Atlas of
Surgical Techniques for the
Upper Gastrointestinal Tract
and Small Bowel

A Volume in the Surgical Techniques Atlas Series

Editor

Michael J. Rosen, MD
Chief, Division of Gastrointestinal and General Surgery
Director, Case Comprehensive Hernia Center
Assistant Professor
Case Medical Center
University Hospitals of Cleveland
Cleveland, Ohio

Jeffrey R. Ponsky, MD
Chairman, Department of Surgery
Case Medical Center
University Hospitals of Cleveland
Cleveland, Ohio

Series Editors

Courtney M. Townsend, Jr., MD
Professor and John Woods Harris Distinguished Chairman
Department of Surgery
The University of Texas Medical Branch
Galveston, Texas

B. Mark Evers, MD
Director, Lucille P. Markey Cancer Center
Professor and Vice-Chair for Research, UK Department of Surgery
Markey Cancer Center Director Chair
Physician-in-Chief, Oncology Service Line
University of Kentucky
Markey Cancer Center
Lexington, Kentucky

SAUNDERS

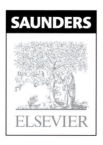

ELSEVIER

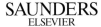
SAUNDERS
ELSEVIER

1600 John F. Kennedy Blvd.
Ste 1800
Philadelphia, PA 19103-2899

ATLAS OF SURGICAL TECHNIQUES FOR THE UPPER GASTROINTESTINAL
TRACT AND SMALL BOWEL   ISBN: 978-1-4160-5278-4

Notice

Knowledge and best practice in this field are constantly changing. As new research and experience broaden our knowledge, changes in practice, treatment and drug therapy may become necessary or appropriate. Readers are advised to check the most current information provided (i) on procedures featured or (ii) by the manufacturer of each product to be administered, to verify the recommended dose or formula, the method and duration of administration, and contraindications. It is the responsibility of the practitioner, relying on their own experience and knowledge of the patient, to make diagnoses, to determine dosages and the best treatment for each individual patient, and to take all appropriate safety precautions. To the fullest extent of the law, neither the Publisher nor the Authors assumes any liability for any injury and/or damage to persons or property arising out of or related to any use of the material contained in this book.

The Publisher

Library of Congress Cataloging-in-Publication Data
Atlas of surgical techniques for the upper gastrointestinal tract and small bowel / editors, Michael J. Rosen, Jeffrey R. Ponsky.—1st ed.
     p. ; cm.—(Surgical techniques atlas series)
  Includes bibliographical references.
  ISBN 978-1-4160-5278-4 (hardcover : alk. paper)
1. Gastrointestinal system–Surgery–Atlases.   2. Intestine, Small–Surgery–Atlases. I. Rosen, Michael J. II. Ponsky, Jeffrey R. III. Series: Surgical techniques atlas series.
  [DNLM: 1. Upper Gastrointestinal Tract–surgery–Atlases. 2. Gastrointestinal Diseases–surgery–Atlases. 3. Intestine, Small–surgery–Atlases. WI 17 A8796 2010]
  RD540.A85 2010
  617.4'300222—dc22

2009029395

Acquisitions Editor: Judith Fletcher
Developmental Editor: Sarah Myer
Publishing Services Manager: Jeff Patterson
Project Manager: Amy Rickles
Design Direction: Steven Stave

Printed in China

Last digit is the print number: 9 8 7 6 5 4 3 2 1

Atlas of
Surgical Techniques for the Upper Gastrointestinal Tract and Small Bowel

Forthcoming Volumes in the Surgical Techniques Atlas Series

Atlas of Endocrine Surgical Techniques
Edited by Quan-Yang Duh, MD, Orlo H. Clark, MD & Electron Kebebew, MD

Atlas of Breast Surgical Techniques
Edited by V. Suzanne Klimberg, MD

Atlas of Thoracic Surgical Techniques
Edited by Joseph B. Zwischenberger, MD

Atlas of Minimally Invasive Surgical Techniques
Edited by Stanley W. Ashley, MD and Ashley Haralson Vernon, MD

Atlas of Pediatric Surgical Techniques
Edited by Dai H. Chung, MD and Mike Kuang Sing Chen, MD

Atlas of Trauma/Emergency Surgical Techniques
Edited by William Cioffi, Jr., MD

Atlas of Surgical Techniques for Colon, Rectum, and Anus
Edited by James W. Fleshman, MD

Atlas of Surgical Techniques for the Hepatobiliary Tract and Pancreas
Edited by Reid B. Adams, MD

CONTRIBUTORS

Alfredo M. Carbonell, DO, FACS, FACOS
Assistant Professor of Clinical Surgery
Division of Minimal Access and Bariatric Surgery
Greenville Hospital System University Medical Center
University of South Carolina School of Medicine
Greenville, South Carolina

Bradley Champagne, MD
Assistant Professor
General Surgery, Division of Colorectal Surgery
Case Medical Center
Cleveland, Ohio

William S. Cobb IV, MD
Associate Professor
Department of Surgery
University of South Carolina School of Medicine
Greenville, South Carolina

Matthew O. Hubbard, MD
Dudley P. Allen Research Fellow
Resident in General Surgery
Department of Surgery
Case Western Reserve University
Case Medical Center
Cleveland, Ohio

Leena Khaitan, MD, MPH
Associate Professor of Surgery
Case Western Reserve University
Cleveland, Ohio
Director of Bariatrics and Minimally Invasive Surgery
Geauga Medical Center
Chardon, Ohio

Julian A. Kim, MD, FACS
Professor and Chief, Surgical Oncology
Department of Surgery
Case Western Reserve University Hospitals
Cleveland, Ohio

Philip A. Linden, MD, FACS, FCCP
Associate Professor of Surgery
Case Western Reserve University
Chief, Division of Thoracic and Esophageal Surgery
Case Medical Center
Cleveland, Ohio

Michael J. Rosen, MD
Chief, Division of Gastrointestinal and General
   Surgery
Director, Case Comprehensive Hernia Center
Assistant Professor
Case Medical Center
University Hospitals of Cleveland
Cleveland, Ohio

FOREWORD

This atlas is for practicing surgeons, surgical residents, and medical students for their review and preparation for surgical procedures. New procedures are developed and old ones are replaced as technologic and pharmacologic advances occur. The topics presented are contemporaneous surgical procedures with step-by-step illustrations, preoperative and postoperative considerations, and pearls and pitfalls, taken from the personal experience and surgical practice of the authors. Their results have been validated in their surgical practices involving many patients. Operative surgery remains a manual art in which the knowledge, judgment, and technical skill of the surgeon come together for the benefit of the patient. A technically perfect operation is the key to this success. Speed in operation comes from having a plan and devoting sufficient time to completion of each step, in order, one time. The surgeon must be dedicated to spending the time to do it right the first time; if not, there will never be enough time to do it right at any other time. Use this atlas; study it for your patients.

Courtney M. Townsend, Jr., MD
B. Mark Evers, MD

PREFACE

Foregut surgery provides the general surgeon the unique ability to treat a multitude of gastrointestinal diseases, including functional disorders of the esophagus, malignancies, morbid obesity, gastroesophageal reflux disease, and peptic ulcer disease. The surgical approaches to these diseases have evolved over the last several years with the rapid influx of minimally invasive techniques. It is important to point out that many disorders of the foregut require complex medical workups and substantial preoperative decision algorithms, which are not covered in this atlas. The atlas of foregut surgery focuses on the technical aspects of gastrointestinal surgery. We have paid particular attention to the operative steps of the respective procedures. We hope to provide a strategy both for avoiding common pitfalls in the operating room and for dealing with technical challenges once they are encountered. In this textbook, both laparoscopic and open approaches are described in detail to allow the surgeon to be comfortable with both techniques and to provide patients with the best outcomes. While there are often many ways to complete a successful operation, this textbook gives examples of safe and effective strategies to dealing with these common problems by various experts in this field. We hope these chapters provide a useful guide to the practicing surgeon in the care of gastrointestinal diseases of the foregut.

Michael Rosen, MD

CONTENTS

Section I Esophagus

CHAPTER 1   TRI-INCISIONAL ESOPHAGECTOMY   1
Philip A. Linden, MD, FACS, FCCP, and Matthew O. Hubbard, MD

CHAPTER 2   IVOR LEWIS ESOPHAGECTOMY   15
Philip A. Linden, MD, FACS, FCCP

CHAPTER 3   LEFT THORACOABDOMINAL   21
Philip A. Linden, MD, FACS, FCCP

CHAPTER 4   TRANSHIATAL   27
Philip A. Linden, MD, FACS, FCCP, and Matthew O. Hubbard, MD

CHAPTER 5   MINIMALLY INVASIVE ESOPHAGECTOMY   33
Philip A. Linden, MD, FACS, FCCP

Section II Hiatal Hernia Surgery

CHAPTER 6   NISSEN FUNDOPLICATION   40
Michael J. Rosen, MD

CHAPTER 7   PARAESOPHAGEAL HERNIA REPAIR   52
Michael J. Rosen, MD

CHAPTER 8   HELLER MYOTOMY   65
Michael J. Rosen, MD

Section III Stomach

CHAPTER 9   TRUNCAL VAGOTOMY   72
Alfredo M. Carbonell, DO, FACS, FACOS

CHAPTER 10   SELECTIVE VAGOTOMY   78
Alfredo M. Carbonell, DO, FACS, FACOS

CHAPTER 11   HIGHLY SELECTIVE VAGOTOMY   82
Alfredo M. Carbonell, DO, FACS, FACOS

CHAPTER 12   HEINEKE-MIKULICZ PYLOROPLASTY   87
William S. Cobb IV, MD

CHAPTER 13   FINNEY PYLOROPLASTY   97
William S. Cobb IV, MD

CHAPTER 14   JABOULAY PYLOROPLASTY   104
William S. Cobb IV, MD

CHAPTER 15   ANTRECTOMY   110
William S. Cobb IV, MD

CHAPTER 16   SURGICAL TREATMENT OF POSTGASTRECTOMY SYNDROMES   127
Alfredo M. Carbonell, DO, FACS, FACOS

CHAPTER 17   LAPAROSCOPIC GASTRIC ULCER SURGERY   137
William S. Cobb IV, MD

Section IV   Gastric Cancer Surgery

CHAPTER 18   SUBTOTAL GASTRECTOMY: BILLROTH I AND II   145
Julian A. Kim, MD, FACS

CHAPTER 19   TOTAL GASTRECTOMY   153
Julian A. Kim, MD, FACS

Section V   Morbid Obesity Surgery

CHAPTER 20   ROUX-EN-Y GASTRIC BYPASS   161
Leena Khaitan, MD, MPH

CHAPTER 21   GASTRIC BAND   177
Leena Khaitan, MD, MPH

CHAPTER 22   GASTRIC SLEEVE   187
Leena Khaitan, MD, MPH

Section VI   Small Intestine Surgery

CHAPTER 23   SMALL BOWEL RESECTION AND ANASTOMOSIS   194
Bradley Champagne, MD

CHAPTER 24   JEJUNOSTOMY TUBE   206
Bradley Champagne, MD

CHAPTER 25   STRICTUROPLASTY FOR CROHN'S DISEASE   213
Bradley Champagne, MD

CHAPTER 26   LAPAROSCOPY FOR CROHN'S DISEASE   218
Bradley Champagne, MD

CHAPTER 27   MECKEL DIVERTICULECTOMY   224
Bradley Champagne, MD

CHAPTER 28   INTUSSCEPTION REDUCTION   228
Bradley Champagne, MD

CHAPTER 29   SMALL BOWEL OBSTRUCTION   231
Bradley Champagne, MD

INDEX   237

CHAPTER 1

TRI-INCISIONAL ESOPHAGECTOMY

Philip A. Linden, MD, FACS, FCCP, and Matthew O. Hubbard, MD

Step 1: Surgical Anatomy

- The normal stomach will reach the neck when placed in situ in virtually every patient. If a patient has had prior gastric surgery, then it may not reach the neck.
- The upper and mid esophagus are most easily accessed via right-side thoracotomy, as the esophagus deviates to the right and there is no intervening aortic arch.
- The azygous vein crosses the esophagus at approximately the junction of the first third and second third of the esophagus. If the azygous vein is unusually large, it should be preserved. The azygous is infrequently a continuation of an interrupted inferior vena cava.
- The left recurrent nerve loops around the aortic arch and ascends in the tracheoesophageal groove in the chest. The right recurrent nerve loops around the right subclavian artery and ascends in the tracheoesophageal groove. Both nerves are best avoided by keeping dissection inside the vagus nerves above the level of the azygous vein.

Step 2: Preoperative Considerations

- A mechanical bowel prep is wise if there is a possibility of requiring a colon interposition instead of a gastric conduit.
- Preoperative intravenous antibiotics are administered. Although many prefer broad spectrum IV antibiotics, there is no data to show that these are superior to preoperative antibiotics directed only at gram-positive organisms.
- All patients undergoing esophagectomy are at high risk of deep vein thrombosis and pulmonary embolism, and they should receive perioperative subcutaneous heparin and sequential compression devices.
- Patients with limited exercise capacity and risk factors for coronary artery disease (CAD) should undergo cardiac testing prior to operation. Patients with a recent change in cardiac symptoms, change in their EKG, possible aortic stenosis, or signs or symptoms of heart failure should also undergo cardiac evaluation.

- Many factors, including location of tumor, extent of dysplasia, surgeon experience, lung and cardiac function, and patient anatomy factor into the route and method of esophagectomy.
- Patients with bulky mid-esophageal tumors, especially those who have undergone neoadjuvant chemoradiation, are best treated with a transthoracic approach.
- Patients with very poor pulmonary function (i.e., FEV_1 <40% predicted) may be better served with a thoracoscopic dissection or transhiatal approach.
- Bronchoscopy with full visualization of the membranous trachea and left main bronchus should be performed by the surgeon for all tumors of the mid and upper esophagus.
- Esophagogastroduodenoscopy must be performed by the surgeon prior to incision.
- A thoracic-level epidural is very useful in managing perioperative pain and minimizing the incidence of pulmonary complications after a thoracotomy.
- The advantages of the tri-incisional esophagectomy include: the complete removal of the esophagus; safe dissection of bulky tumors in the chest under direct vision; and an anastomosis out of the chest.
- Disadvantages include the need for a chest incision, and the higher incidence of recurrent nerve injury with a neck anastomosis.
- Patients with tumors at or above the level of the carina generally require a tri-incisional approach with an anastomosis in the neck.

Step 3: Operative Steps

1. Right Thoracotomy

- The patient is placed in the left lateral decubitus position with an approximate 30-degree forward tilt.
- An abbreviated right posterolateral thoracotomy is performed, starting beneath the tip of the scapula and extending posteriorly 10 cm—typically just long enough to allow introduction of the surgeon's hand.
- The latissimus is divided and the serratus muscle is spared and retracted anteriorly. Entry into the chest is on top of the sixth rib, in the fifth interspace. A 2-cm-long portion of the posterior sixth rib is removed to facilitate spreading of the ribs. The lung is retracted anteriorly and the inferior pulmonary ligament is divided with cautery.
- Starting at a region in the esophagus away from the tumor, the pleura is incised just anterior to the azygous vein. Posterior dissection is performed with a large, blunt right-angle or Harken #1 clamp. Medially, the pleural reflection is taken off the pericardium and dissection proceeds posteriorly. Dissection continues with cautery until a finger can encircle the esophagus, followed by a Penrose drain. All tissue lateral to the pericardium is included in the specimen. (Figure 1-1)
- For tumors at the GE junction, one may choose first to perform dissection in a cranial direction. To the right of the esophagus, all tissue medial to the azygous vein is included in the specimen—branches from the aorta are clipped on the aortic side, and cauterized on the esophageal side. All tissue is dissected off the pericardium and included in the specimen. The Penrose drain is used to distract the specimen away from surrounding tissue.
- On the left, the esophagus is dissected off the pericardium, and then away from the left main bronchus. On the right and posteriorly the esophagus is dissected off the aorta, clipping all large branches.
- The anterior vagus nerve is divided at this level, and dissection proceeds in between the vagus nerve and esophagus. (Figure 1-2)
- The posterior (left) vagus nerve is also identified and dissected away from the esophagus.

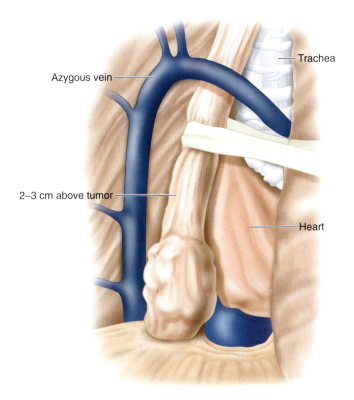

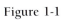

Figure 1-1

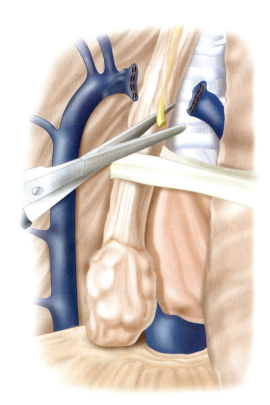

Figure 1-2

- The azygous vein is divided with an endovascular 2.5-mm stapler.
- Using low cautery settings, the esophagus is dissected away from the carina and trachea. Some of the dissection may be done using blunt finger dissection.
- The apical portion of mediastinal pleura is preserved in order to minimize the risk of contamination from a cervical leak.
- Dissection at the thoracic inlet is performed bluntly with the fingertip, preserving the apical pleura.
- The Penrose drain is knotted and placed along the cervical spine for retrieval during the cervical phase of the operation.
- Another Penrose drain is placed around the esophagus, and dissection proceeds in a caudal direction.
- Medial dissection removes the esophagus and periesophageal tissue off the pericardium.
- The esophagus is dissected laterally away from the aorta and azygous vein. Large arterial feeders should be clipped on the aortic side.
- Extensive dissection to the right and posterior to the esophagus enters the region of the thoracic duct, but must be performed for bulky tumors.
- For GE-junction tumors, a rim of diaphragm is included in the specimen. The rim is elevated away from intraabdominal structures using a large right-angle clamp.
- Mass ligation of the thoracic duct is performed at the level of the esophageal hiatus.
  - ▲ The pleura overlying the vertebral body lateral to the aorta is incised.
  - ▲ A blunt-tipped right-angle is used to encircle all tissue anterior to the vertebral body and aorta.
  - ▲ A #1 silk ligature is used to tie the tissue; take care not to tie too tightly, which could tear through the duct. (Figure 1-3)
  - ▲ A suture ligature can be performed, but there may be a higher risk of lacerating the duct.
- The Penrose is knotted and placed into the abdomen for retrieval during the abdominal phase of the operation.
- An examination of the esophageal bed is made for bleeding or for leakage of clear fluid, which may be an indication of a thoracic duct tear in the unfed patient.
- A 28 straight chest tube is placed to the right apex with an additional hole cut to drain fluid from the right pleural base.
- The chest is closed with #1 or #2 Vicryl paracostal sutures.
- Latissimus is reapproximated with a running 0 Vicryl suture.
- The subdermal layer is closed with a running 2-0 Vicryl suture.
- The subcuticular layer is closed with a running 3-0 monocryl or Vicryl suture.

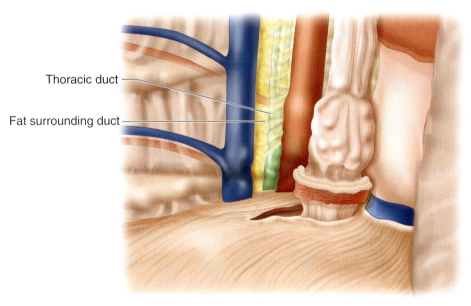

Thoracic duct

Fat surrounding duct

Figure 1-3

2. Laparotomy

- A midline upper laparotomy is performed from the base of the xiphoid process to 2 cm above the umbilicus. If the xiphoid process is excessively large, it can be excised.
- The omentum, liver, and serosal surfaces of the abdomen are explored for metastatic disease. If preoperative suspicion of abdominal metastatic disease is high, as in patients with celiac adenopathy, minimal response to neoadjuvant therapy, or signet cell pathology, a laparoscopy should be performed as the initial step. The right gastroepiploic artery is palpated—the pulse should be strong.
- An upper hand retractor is placed at about the level of the nipples. A Balfour retractor is used in addition to the upper hand retractor. Alternatively an Omni-type retractor can be used as the sole retractor. The patient is placed in a reverse Trendelenburg position.
- The attachments between the left lobe of the liver and the diaphragm are divided, taking care not to injure the left hepatic vein. The left lobe of the liver can be folded downward and retracted if the lobe is thin, taking care not to lacerate the surface of the liver. If the left lobe of the liver is thick, then it should be elevated anteriorly.
- Cautery is used to enter and divide the clear areas of the gastrohepatic ligament. An ultrasonic scalpel can be used for thicker areas of the ligament. Dissection proceeds up to the right crus.
- If a Penrose drain has been placed during the thoracic phase of the operation, it is now located and grasped. If not, a rim of diaphragm is included with the esophagus at the hiatus, with care to suture ligate the phrenic vein, which crosses anteriorly.
- At approximately the midpoint of greater curvature, entry is made into the lesser sac, several centimeters away from the gastroepiploic artery. Cranial dissection proceeds with cautery through clear areas, and with ultrasonic scalpel or with clamping and ligation through areas with thicker tissue. The surgeon to the patient's right side grasps the greater curvature of the stomach (with care not to compress or manipulate the right gastroepiploic artery) and retracts medially. The surgeon to the patient's left side uses one hand to keep abdominal contents away from the area of dissection and the other hand to distract tissue laterally.
- Dissection proceeds along the greater curvature with care to stay at least 2 cm away from the gastroepiploic artery. The artery eventually ends, and the lateral arcades supplying the stomach become short gastric arteries.
- The anterior and posterior leafs of the short gastrics may be divided with the ultrasonic scalpel, or may be divided with sequential firings of the endoscopic stapler (2.0-mm-thick staples). Often the highest short gastrics enter the cardia of the stomach immediately adjacent to the left crus. Dissection into the splenic artery or pancreas must be avoided. Dense adhesions in this area may make dissection difficult.
- Typically there are loose adhesions between the posterior aspects of the stomach and pancreas, which are divided with cautery.
- The stomach is retracted anteriorly, and the pedicle of the left gastric artery is identified. Sharp dissection with blunt-tip scissors or with cautery is used to dissect all nodes at the origin of the left gastric artery and sweep them onto the specimen. Celiac nodes can also be dissected in this fashion. (Figure 1-4) The base of the left gastric artery is clamped with an endovascular stapler that is 45 mm in length and 2.5 mm in height. The right gastroepiploic artery should be palpated at this point to insure that the celiac axis has not been clamped and the stapler is fired. (Figure 1-5)
- At this point dissection proceeds along the greater curvature of the stomach toward the pylorus. The gastroepiploic artery may wander away from the greater curvature of the stomach in this location.
- A Kocher maneuver is performed by retracting all abdominal contents to the patient's left side. Any adhesions between the gallbladder and duodenum are lysed. The duodenum is found at the pylorus and followed to where it attaches to the retroperitoneum. The highest peritoneal attachments are incised with scissors. The surgeon's index finger may then be introduced behind the lateral attachments, and cautery on the index finger will release the attachments. Gentle blunt sweeping of the duodenum medially can be performed with the surgeon's finger or a sponge stick. The medial blood supply to the duodenum must be preserved.

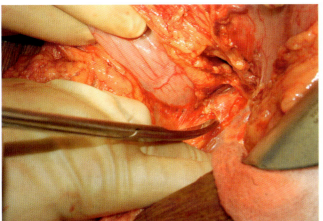

Figure 1-4

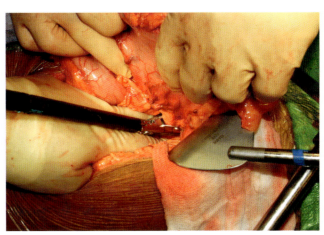

Figure 1-5

3. Cervical and Laparotomy Phase

- An incision is made from the sternal notch to the level of the cricoid cartilage, anterior to the border of the left sternocleidomastoid muscle (about 6 cm). The platysma is divided with cautery. The omohyoid may be divided with cautery if it interferes with access to the esophagus.
- A self-retaining retractor may be used, but the medial blades should be placed against the skin and platysma, and must not rest in the tracheoesophageal groove.
- Blunt dissection is performed with the two index fingers medial to the jugular sheath and lateral to the trachea down to the vertebral body. The prevertebral plane is entered, the knot in the Penrose drain is palpated, and the Penrose drain is brought up into the wound.
- Additional gentle blunt dissection may be performed to obtain additional proximal length on the esophagus.
- The nasogastric tube is withdrawn, a GIA stapler (35-mm height) is applied across the esophagus, and a heavy, 36-inch stitch is attached to the specimen side. The stapler is fired, and the specimen and stitch are brought into the abdomen. A snap is placed on the end of the suture remaining in the neck.
- A snap is placed on the end of the suture in the abdomen.
- At a point on the lesser curvature near the crow's foot of veins, the right gastric artery and surrounding tissue are dissected free and ligated or divided with an endovascular stapler.
- The gastric tube is created: At a point on the greater curvature approximately 6 cm from the edge of tumor, thick-tissue (48 mm in height) GIA 80-mm staplers are applied parallel to the greater curvature of the stomach. A conduit width of at least 5 cm is desirable to allow for adequate conduit emptying. (Figure 1-6)
- Care is taken to insure that excess gastric tissue does not "bunch-up" in the stapler; excess room is left at each end of the stapler during each fire. Sequential firings of the thick-tissue stapler are performed taking care to align the staple lines. Three to five firings may be needed. (Figure 1-7)
- At this point in time, the specimen is sent to pathology for margins.
- The overlapping areas of the thick-tissue stapler firings on the lesser curve of the stomach are oversewn with imbricating 3-0 silk sutures. Large short gastric stumps are tied with 3-0 silk ties, with care not to incorporate the gastric wall.

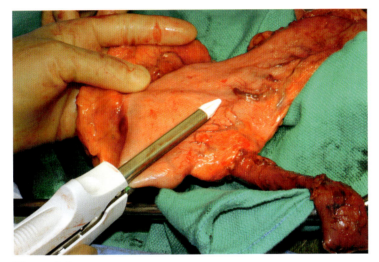

Figure 1-6

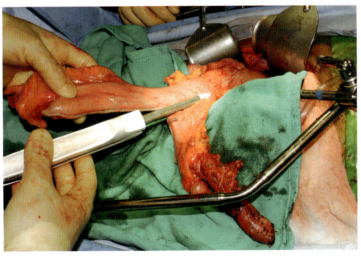

Figure 1-7

- A pyloroplasty or pyloromyotomy, is performed at this point, if the surgeon chooses so. Some surgeons prefer a pyloromyotomy, but are prepared to convert to a pyloroplasty if the lumen is entered. If a pyloroplasty is performed, a right angle clamp is used to elevate the anterior portion of the gastric and duodenal wall away from the posterior wall aids in visualizing the mucosa and in avoiding closing the anterior and posterior walls together.
- Prior to bringing the conduit into the chest and neck, inspection for hemostasis is made in the bed of the mobilized stomach.
- One atraumatic method of bringing the conduit into the neck involves an endoscopic camera bag. A 30-cc Foley balloon is placed into a laparoscopic camera bag, and the bag is tied around the Foley using heavy silk suture. The balloon is filled with saline. The long heavy silk ligature traversing the chest is attached to the valved end of the Foley and is brought into the neck.
- The conduit is placed into the bag, properly oriented so that the staple line is on the patient's right side. Suction is applied to the drainage port of the Foley and the assistant draws the Foley up into the neck. The surgeon on the right side of the abdomen grasps the bag containing the tip of the conduit and guides it up into the chest, until the pylorus lies at the hiatus. (Figures 1-8 and 1-9)
- The bag is opened in the neck and a Babcock instrument is used to grasp the tip of the stomach.
- A corner of the esophageal staple line is cut off with scissors. Cautery is used to make a 1-cm hole in the gastric conduit opposite the staple line. The entrance into the gastric conduit should be placed at a distance from the staple line to minimize ischemia.
- One limb of a GIA 80 mm 35 mm in height stapler is placed in the esophagus and the other limb is placed into the gastric lumen. The stapler is fired to create the anastomosis. As the stapler is separated and withdrawn, the staple line is inspected for hemostasis. The nasogastric tube is passed with its tip verified at the pylorus, and the enterotomy site is closed with either 3-0 interrupted silk sutures or a TA 60 thick-tissue stapler. (Figure 1-10ABC)
- A Penrose or JP drain is placed posteriorly along the spine, and the platysma is closed with interrupted suture. The skin is closed with staples.
- After the creation of a J-tube, the abdomen is closed with running looped #1 PDS or Prolene and staples for the skin.

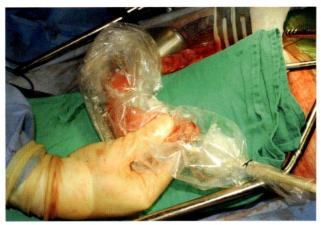

Figure 1-8

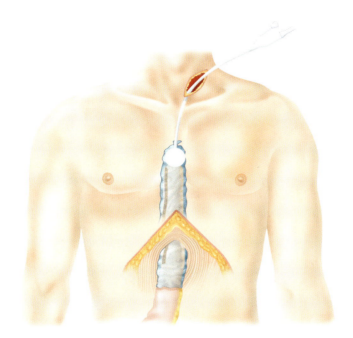

Figure 1-9

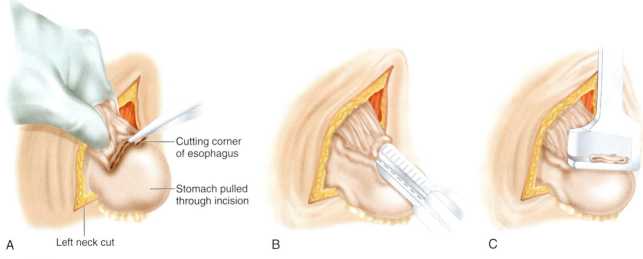

A   Left neck cut

Cutting corner
of esophagus

Stomach pulled
through incision

B

C

Figure 1-10

Step 4: Postoperative Care

- The chest tube can be removed when the drainage is about 200 cc per day, usually by postoperative day 2 or 3. There is little merit to leaving the chest tubes in until a swallowing study is done—intrathoracic leaks generally require immediate reoperation.
- The epidural is generally left in place until after the chest tube is removed and the patient is tolerating enteral narcotics (typically 5 to 6 days).
- Typical presenting symptoms of chyle leaks are high chest tube output (500 cc to 1 L or more per day) that persists after postoperative day (POD) 2. The fluid may be clear but turns milky white after feeding the patient with several hundred mls of heavy cream via J-tube. Treatment is mandatory. If the duct is found to be large during an MRI, then percutaneous fenestration and/or coiling of the duct is an effective treatment. Reoperation with mass ligation (or re-ligation) of the duct at the hiatus and suture of the duct injury with fine Prolene and pledgets is the standard treatment. Instilling 200 cc of cream into the J-tube several hours prior to the operation helps with identifying the site of the leak.
- The neck drain is typically left until after the swallow is performed. A barium swallow will miss 10% of cervical leaks. The patient is then asked to drink grape juice (its purple color is not confused with serosanguineous drainage). If no purple fluid is seen in the drain, then it is removed.
- Recent publications have shown that the pulmonary complications are the main contributors to mortality following esophagectomy.
- One must be vigilant to recognize recurrent nerve injuries. These typically present with hoarseness or a soft voice, and an ineffective cough. This may not present until postoperative day 2 or 3 when cord swelling from double lumen tube intubation and fluid administration subsides. A patient with a recurrent nerve injury may also be at increased risk of aspiration. Immediate medialization of the cord (usually by injection) will improve the voice and cough and allow for effective clearance of pulmonary secretions. Occasionally, a patient with a recurrent nerve injury may still have an effective cough. If so, treatment may be deferred if a video swallow shows no increased risk of aspiration.
- Patients undergoing esophagectomy are at extremely high risk for DVT and PE. They should have sequential pneumatic compression boots applied and subcutaneous heparin administered upon induction of anesthesia.
- Postoperative hypotension is not uncommon, especially with the use of epidurals, and should be treated with aggressive and generous volume administration and not pressors. Generally by postoperative day 2-3 intravenous fluids can be stopped and diuresis begun.
- Extreme vigilance must be maintained for signs or symptoms of conduit necrosis or leak. Unexplained fever, tachycardia, leukocytosis, or pleural effusion should raise suspicion. A base deficit can be a sign of conduit hypoperfusion, but is nonspecific and common after esophagectomy for the first 12 to 24 hours.
- Patients should be maintained with the head of bed elevated 30 degrees or greater to minimize the risk of aspiration pneumonia.
- Ambulation starting on POD1 helps prevent DVT and speeds recovery. Epidurals, chest tubes, oxygen, and Foley catheters should not anchor a patient to their bed.
- Low-dose beta blockade (metoprolol 5 mg IV q4h) is useful in preventing atrial fibrillation, and in controlling the rate should fibrillation occur.
- Tube feeds are begun after flatus at 30 cc per hour at full strength and advanced at 10 cc/hr every 12 hours. Some choose to begin tube feeds prior to evidence of return of bowel function, with care to watch for abdominal distension and avoid ileus with duodenal distension. An ileus in an esophagectomy patient can easily lead to aspiration pneumonia.
- Patients are typically discharged on full liquid diets for 1 to 2 weeks until anastomotic swelling resolves. They can then advance to soft solid food.

Step 5: Pearls and Pitfalls

- At the level of the azygous vein, the vagus nerves should be identified and detached from the esophagus. Cranial dissection proceeds within the vagus nerves.
- Cautery must be done carefully along the course of the trachea and at low settings in order to avoid delayed tracheoesophageal fistula or left recurrent nerve injury.
- During mobilization of the stomach, the surgeon must be vigilant about preservation of the gastroepiploic vascular arcade. Excessive handling, manual compression, thermal injury, and suture injury can turn a routine operation into a life-threatening event. In the obese patient the artery may be difficult to see and its location should be continually reassessed.
- The highest and largest short gastric arteries should be tied on the gastric side in order to avoid postoperative bleeding. It is usually easiest to do this after completion of the gastric tube after initially dividing the short gastrics with an ultrasonic scalpel. Simple use of an ultrasonic scalpel or clips may be inadequate. The ties must not incorporate gastric wall—delayed necrosis and perforation may result.
- Unlike most applications of staplers, the creation of the gastric tube with the GIA thick-tissue stapler requires great care. Excess tissue must not bunch up into the stapler. Successive applications of the stapler should be carefully aligned. The point of intersection of successive staple lines should be imbricated with silk sutures.
- When the conduit is passed through the chest up into the neck, it must be guided through the hiatus from below. Correct orientation must be insured so that the conduit does not twist 180 degrees.

References

1. McKeown KC. Total three-stage oesophagectomy for cancer of the oesophagus. *Br J Surg* 1976; 63:259.
2. Linden PA, Sugarbaker DJ. Esophagectomy via right thoracotomy. In: Patterson GA, et al, eds. *Pearson's thoracic and esophageal surgery*. 3rd ed. Philadelphia: Churchill Livingstone Elsevier; 2008.
3. Swanson SJ, Batierel HF, Bueno R, et al. Transthoracic esophagectomy with radical mediastinal and abdominal lymph node dissection and cervical esophagogastrotomy for esophageal carcinoma. *Ann Thorac Surg* 2001; 72:1918-1925.

CHAPTER 2

Ivor Lewis Esophagectomy

Philip A. Linden, MD, FACS, FCCP

Step 1: Surgical Anatomy

- The azygous vein crosses the esophagus at approximately the junction of the first third and second third of the esophagus. If the azygous vein is unusually large, it should be preserved. The azygous is infrequently a continuation of an interrupted inferior vena cava.
- The lower esophagus is a left-sided structure. Access from the right chest is possible but is difficult from a high right thoracotomy. Dissection of the hiatus and lower esophagus is best performed during the abdominal phase of this operation.

Step 2: Preoperative Considerations

- See Chapter 1 for general preoperative considerations.
- Patients with bulky mid-esophageal tumors, especially who have undergone neoadjuvant chemoradiation, are best treated with a transthoracic approach.
- Patients with very poor pulmonary function (i.e., FEV_1 <40% predicted) may be better served with a thoracoscopic dissection or transhiatal approach.
- The advantages of the Ivor Lewis approach include the direct dissection of a tumor in the chest, good nodal clearance, and less chance for recurrent nerve injury than with a cervical incision.
- Disadvantages include the need for a thoracotomy, life-threatening sepsis that may accompany an anastomotic leak, and a proximal margin that is approximately 3 cm shorter than with a cervical incision.

Step 3: Operative Steps

1. Laparotomy and Gastric Mobilization

- The entire stomach is dissected as described under "laparotomy" in Chapter 1.
- A complete Kocher maneuver is performed, including lysis of any adhesions between the gallbladder and duodenum.

- If a T2 (by endoscopic ultrasound [EUS]), or higher, tumor is present, a rim of diaphragm is now incised and included on the specimen. For T1 or intramucosal tumors, it is acceptable to dissect between the hiatus and esophagus.
- Dissection continues in to the lower chest as with a transhiatal dissection. The harmonic scalpel is an ideal instrument to use during this portion of the dissection. The esophagus is distracted anteriorly during posterior dissection, to the right during dissection on the left, and to the left for dissection on the right.
- A pyloroplasty or pyloromyotomy is performed at this point, if at all.
- The conduit may at this point be placed into the right chest for retrieval during the chest phase of the operation. If so, tacking sutures should be placed on the underside of the diaphragm.
  - ▲ The nasogastric tube is withdrawn. The gastric tube may be created in the abdomen by firing an endovascular stapler across the right gastric artery near the crow's foot of veins. Sequential firings of a GIA 4.8 mm in height, 80 mm in length stapler are applied starting at the lesser curvature. Care is taken not to overlap staple lines or include too much tissue in a single firing. The staple line is extended to the cardia of the greater curvature, leaving 6 cm of gross margins.
  - ▲ The section of staple line where stapler firings overlap is reinforced with interrupted, imbricating 3-0 silk sutures.
  - ▲ The mobilized stomach is passed into the chest for later retrieval.
  - ▲ If a gastric tube has been created during the abdominal portion of the operation, it is sutured with heavy 0 sutures to the staple line of the specimen, which includes the distal esophagus and cardia of stomach.
- A J-tube is constructed, and the abdomen is closed.

2. Right Thoracotomy

- The patient is positioned in the left lateral decubitus position. A posterolateral thoracotomy is performed. The latissimus is divided and the serratus spared. Entry into the chest is through the fourth interspace; the fifth rib is shingled posteriorly.
- At a place in the esophagus remote from the tumor, the esophagus is encircled with a Penrose drain.
- Traction is placed on the Penrose opposite the area of esophageal dissection.
- To the right of the esophagus, all tissue medial to the azygous vein is included in the specimen—branches from the aorta are clipped on the aortic side, and cauterized on the esophageal side. All tissue is dissected of the pericardium and included in the specimen. The Penrose is used to distract the specimen away from surrounding tissue.
- On the left, the esophagus is dissected off the pericardium, and then away from the left main bronchus. On the right and posteriorly the esophagus is dissected off the aorta, clipping all large branches.
- The anterior vagus nerve is divided at this level and dissection proceeds in between the vagus nerve and esophagus.
- The posterior (left) vagus nerve is also identified and dissected away from the esophagus.
- The azygous vein is divided with an endovascular 2.5-mm stapler.
- The upper line of the division is chosen, usually at the level of the divided azygous vein. Minimal dissection of the esophagus is performed above the planned area of division. The gastric conduit is brought into the chest. If the gastric tube has not yet been created, then it is fashioned at this point.

- The length of gastric conduit should be estimated. If there is excess length, the conduit should be trimmed so that the redundant conduit will not kink in the lower chest.
  - ▲ The anastomosis may be performed using a 25-mm or 28-mm EEA stapler. The upper esophagus is divided with a 3.5-mm stapler, and the staple line is removed. The Λ 2-0 Prolene is used to secure the anvil in the esophagus. Additional stitches may be used to secure the circumferential suture line. The tip of the gastric conduit is removed, and the handle is inserted into the enterotomy. At a comfortable point on the greater curvature of the tube (opposite the staple line), the handle is united with the anvil, and the stapler is fired. (Figure 2-1)
- The anastomosis is checked for leaks by placing the anastomosis under sterile saline and insufflating with the gastroscope.
- A two-layered, hand-sewn anastomosis may also be performed. The point of anastomosis in the gastric conduit is chosen several centimeters away from the lesser curvature staple line. A circumferential incision in the serosa is made, approximately 3 cm in diameter. The underlying submucosal vessels are individually ligated with 3-0 silk sutures. The back wall of the anastomosis is constructed with 3-0 horizontal mattress sutures. Horizontal mattress sutures hold better than simple sutures as the esophagus has no true serosal coating. The posterior half of the esophagus is opened sharply, and a full thickness inner layer is performed with either running or interrupted 4-0 monocryl suture. After completion of the back wall of the inner sutures, the nasogastric tube is passed, the remaining esophagus is divided, and the front portion of the inner anastomosis is completed. The anterior outer layer is completed using 3-0 silk horizontal mattress sutures. (Figure 2-2)
- The anastomosis is buttressed with omentum. Some surgeons choose to tack the conduit to the pleura, though it is not clear if this is necessary.
- Two small 19F Blake drains are placed alongside the anastomosis. A 28F chest tube is placed to the apex. The ribs are approximated with 4 to 6 #2 Vicryl sutures. The latissimus layer is closed using a running 0 Vicryl. The subdermal layer is closed using a running 2-0 Vicryl. The skin is closed using a running subcuticular 3-0 Vicryl or monocryl.

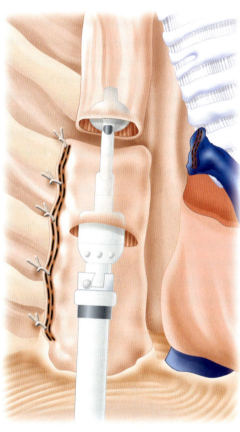
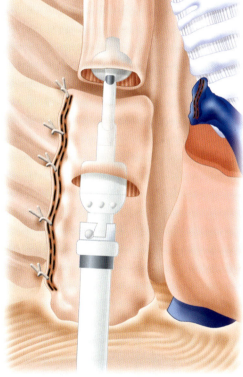
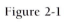

Figure 2-1

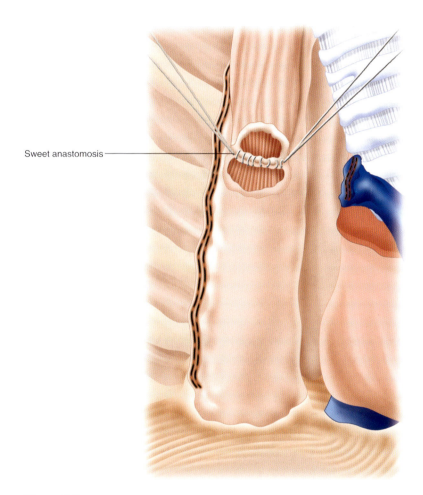

Sweet anastomosis

Figure 2-2

Step 4: Postoperative Care

- Postoperative care is similar to that required for other transthoracic esophageal resections (see Chapter 1).
- One must be vigilant for anastomotic leaks that may present as fever, elevated white blood cell count, hypotension, confusion, or purulent chest tube drainage.
- An intrathoracic leak should prompt an immediate return to the operating room for repair.
- The Blake drains are removed after a negative swallow on postoperative day 6 or 7.

Step 5: Pearls and Pitfalls

- As much dissection as possible of the hiatus and into the lower chest should be performed from the abdomen, as this area is difficult to reach from a fourth interspace thoracotomy.
- There should be minimal dissection of the esophagus above the point of transection, in order to preserve its blood supply.
- Careful handling is required of the tissues that are to be anastomosed. If a hand-sewn anastomosis is performed, one must be certain that each inner stitch is full thickness containing mucosa. They should be placed no more than 2 to 3 mm apart.
- If one is concerned about an intrathoracic leak, sending the adjacent Blake drain contents for amylase may help detect a leak and prompt an early swallow study.
- Prior to construction of the anastomosis, the length of gastric conduit should be inspected. If there is redundant stomach in the chest it may kink in the future leading to difficulties with gastric emptying. It should be trimmed prior to the creation of the anastomosis.

References

1. Chu K, Law S, Wong J, et al. A prospective randomized comparison of transhiatal and transthoracic resection for lower-third esophageal carcinoma. *Am J Surg* 1997; 174:320-324.
2. Churchill ED, Sweet RH: Transthoracic resection of tumors of the stomach and esophagus. *Ann Surg* 1942; 115:897.
3. Ellis FH, Gibb SP, Watkins E Jr. Esophagogastrectomy: A safe, widely applicable and expeditious form of palliation for patients with carcinoma of the esophagus and cardia. *Ann Surg* 1983; 198;531.
4. Goldminc M, Maddern G, LePrise E, et al. Oesophagectomy by a transhiatal approach or thoracotomy: a prospective randomized trial. *Br J Surg* 1993; 80:367-376.
5. Hulscher J, Tijssen J, Lanschot J. Transthoracic versus transhiatal resection for carcinoma of the esophagus: a meta-analysis. *Ann Thor Surg* 2001; 72:306-313.
6. Hulscher J, Van Sandick J, Van Lanschot J. Extended transthoracic resection compared with limited transhiatal resection for adenocarcinoma of the esophagus. *N Engl J Med* 2002; 347:1662-1669.
7. Lewis I. The surgical treatment of carcinoma of the oesophagus with special reference to a new operation for growths of the middle third. *Br J Surg* 1946; 34:18.
8. Mathieson DH, Grillo HC, et al. Transthoracic esophagectomy: a safe approach to carcinoma of the esophagus. *Ann Thorac Surg* 1988; 45:137.
9. Rindani R, Martin C, Cox M. Transhiatal versus Ivor-Lewis oesophagectomy: is there a difference? *Aust N Z J Surg* 1999; 69:187-194.

CHAPTER 3

LEFT THORACOABDOMINAL

Philip A. Linden, MD, FACS, FCCP

Step 1: Surgical Anatomy

- The lower portion of the esophagus deviates to the left of the midline and is most easily accessible via the left chest.
- Above the level of the inferior pulmonary vein, the esophagus deviates to the right, but can still be accessed through the left chest.
- The aortic arch obscures the esophagus when approached through the left chest, but the esophagus can still be mobilized, albeit with more difficulty than via a right thoracotomy.
- The thoracic duct runs behind the junction of the subclavian artery and aortic arch when viewed from the left side and must be avoided.

Step 2: Preoperative Considerations

- See Chapter 1 for general preoperative considerations.
- Patients with very poor pulmonary function (i.e., FEV1 <40% predicted) may be better served with a thoracoscopic dissection or transhiatal approach.
- This approach is useful for tumors of the GE junction and cardia of the stomach. Access to mid and upper third esophageal tumors is much more difficult with this approach, and a tri-incisional approach is preferred.
- The left thoracoabdominal approach allows for simultaneous access to the chest, abdomen, and neck from a single (right lateral decubitus) position.
- This approach is especially useful for GE junction tumors that may have significant extension into both the esophagus and cardia of the stomach. If the stomach margins are positive, a complete gastrectomy with Roux-en-Y anastomosis in the lower chest may be performed. If the esophageal margins are positive, then the stomach may be pulled up into the neck. Complete removal of the stomach and esophagus requires a colon interposition, as Roux-en-Y jejunum generally does not reach into the neck.
- This approach provides for the best visualization of the celiac axis and short gastric vessels.
- Ability to tolerate single lung ventilation is not an absolute requirement as the lower lobe can be mobilized and retracted upward for an anastomosis in the lower chest. Patients with such poor lung function, however, may have fewer pulmonary complications with a transhiatal or thoracoscopic approach.

Step 3: Operative Steps

- The patient is placed in the right lateral decubitus position with the hips rotated about 30 degrees posteriorly.
- A posterolateral thoracotomy incision is made, extending from just behind the tip of the scapula coursing down the seventh interspace. The incision may be stopped at the costal margin, or extended across the costal margin toward the linea alba. Most of the dissection and gastric mobilization can be performed through a generous incision in the diaphragm parallel to the chest wall. The decision to extend the incision across the costal margin and onto the abdomen is based upon the need to perform a Kocher maneuver or pyloroplasty, and any associated abdominal pathology. Some surgeons routinely extend the incision across the costal margin as it makes the dissection easier. (Figure 3-1)
- An incision is made in the diaphragm, 2 to 3 cm away from the diaphragm's insertion site in the chest wall. The diaphragm can be taken down with cautery while being elevated with a large right angle clamp to protect intraabdominal structures. Marking sutures should be placed in both sides of the diaphragm as it is divided to allow for realignment during closure. Alternatively, a 3.5-mm thickness stapler can be used. The sites of intersection of stapler fires aids in realignment of the diaphragm when closing. (Figure 3-2)
- If the decision is made to extend the incision across the costal margin into the abdomen, then the attachment of the diaphragm is bluntly cleared away from the site of division of the costal margin first. The margin is divided with a rib shear, and the takedown of the diaphragm begins at this location.
- A rim of diaphragm is resected along with gastroesophageal junction.
- The lower esophagus is dissected and encircled with a Penrose drain.
- The dissection of gastric conduit is identical to that performed via laparotomy except for a few aspects. The dissection typically begins at the highest short gastrics and proceeds down the greater curvature of the stomach. Care must be taken to notice the onset of the gastroepiploic artery.
- Loose adhesions between the pancreas and posterior stomach are divided with cautery.
- The left gastric artery is easily visualized from this approach. Lymph nodes overlying the artery at its base are swept onto the specimen using sharp dissection, and the base of the artery is divided with an endovascular (2.5-mm thickness) stapler.
- The gastrohepatic ligament is divided with a combination of ultrasonic scalpel (through thick areas) and cautery (through thin areas).
- If the anastomosis is to be made in the lower chest (below the level of the inferior pulmonary vein), then typically a Kocher maneuver is not needed, and the right gastric artery is not divided.

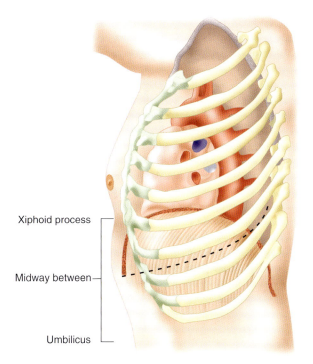

Xiphoid process

Midway between

Umbilicus

Figure 3-1

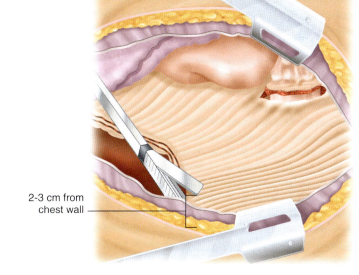

2-3 cm from
chest wall

Figure 3-2

- The esophagus is dissected proximally off the aorta, clipping any large branches. The other borders of the dissection are the pericardium and right pleura, which is often included in the specimen. Proximal dissection is performed with the aim of obtaining a 5- to 6-cm proximal margin.
- The gastric conduit is created as described in Chapter 1, Tri-Incisional Esophagectomy. If the conduit is to be mobilized only to the lower chest, then the right gastric artery may be preserved. If tension is present after mobilization into the chest, then it is divided. (Figure 3-3)
- The anastomosis in the chest may be performed as previously described (hand-sewn anastomosis or EEA in Chapter 2, Ivor Lewis Esophagectomy). A side-to-side, functional end-to-end stapled anastomosis may also be performed as described in Chapter 1. (Figure 3-4)
- If dissection is done behind the aortic arch, care must be taken to avoid injury to the recurrent laryngeal nerve and thoracic duct. After completion of the anastomosis, it is covered with omentum.
- The gastric conduit is tacked circumferentially to the diaphragmatic hiatus with 2-0 absorbable sutures.
- The diaphragm is then reattached to its insertion on the chest wall with interrupted horizontal mattress large sutures (such as 0 silk).
- The costal margin is reapproximated with a figure of eight #1 Prolene.
- The abdomen may be closed with a either a single layer of #1 or #2 PDS or Prolene, or by separate posterior and anterior fascia layers.
- The chest is then closed with interrupted #2 Vicryl paracostal sutures, running 0 Vicryl serratus—latissimus layers, running 2-0 Vicryl subdermal layers, and running 3-0 or 4-0 monocryl subcuticular layers.

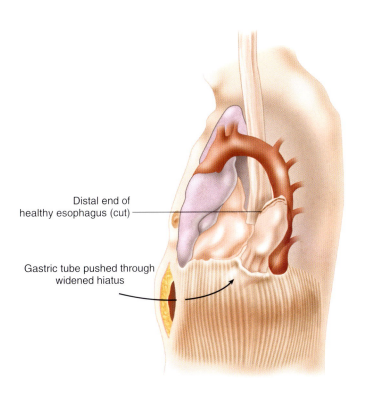

Distal end of
healthy esophagus (cut)

Gastric tube pushed through
widened hiatus

Figure 3-3

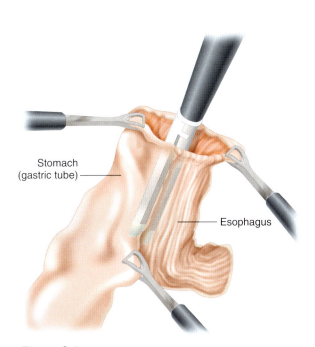

Stomach
(gastric tube)

Esophagus

Figure 3-4

Step 4: Postoperative Care

- Extubation may be performed in the operating room, or it may be deferred if there are concerns with pain control, borderline pulmonary status, large intraoperative fluid requirement, or hemodynamic instability. Bronchoscopy should be performed prior to extubation.
- Postoperative care is similar to that required for other transthoracic esophageal resections (see Chapter 1).
- One must be vigilant for anastomotic leaks, which may present as fever, elevated white blood cell count, hypotension, confusion, or purulent chest tube drainage.
- An intrathoracic leak should prompt an immediate return to the operating room for repair.
- The Blake drains are removed after a negative swallow on postoperative day 6 or 7.

Step 5: Pearls and Pitfalls

- When the diaphragm is taken down from its lateral attachments to the chest wall, at least 2 cm should be left on the chest wall. This will aid in closure of the diaphragm.
- A peripheral incision in the diaphragm will spare branches of the phrenic nerve and retain diaphragmatic function.
- The costal margin site of division is at risk of poor healing and chronic pain. The margin can be divided sharply with electrocautery or a rib shear, and should be reapproximated carefully using a heavy, nonabsorbable suture such as #1 Prolene.
- As one proceeds with dissection of the greater curvature starting at the short gastrics and progressing toward the pylorus, one must be careful to notice the onset of the gastroepiploic artery and dissect at least 2 cm lateral to the artery.
- If one has to mobilize the esophagus behind the aortic arch, one should be careful not to injure the thoracic duct, which courses behind the subclavian artery. Routine ligation of the region of the thoracic duct at the diaphragmatic should be done if dissection is carried out behind the arch.

References

1. Ginsberg R. Left thoracoabdominal cervical approach. In: Pearson FG, ed. *Esophageal surgery*. 2nd ed. Philadelphia: Churchill Livingstone; 2002.
2. Linden P, Swanson S. Esophageal resection and replacement. In: Sellke F, del Nido P, Swanson S, eds. *Sabiston and Spencer surgery of the chest*. 7th ed. Philadelphia: Elsevier Saunders; 2005.

4

TRANSHIATAL

Philip A. Linden, MD, FACS, FCCP, and Matthew O. Hubbard, MD

Step 1: Surgical Anatomy

- Patients with bulky mid-esophageal tumors, especially those who have undergone neoadjuvant chemoradiation, are best treated with a transthoracic approach.
- The transhiatal approach is useful for patients with poor lung function (FEV$_1$ <1 liter or <50% predicted).
- Fewer lymph nodes are harvested with a transhiatal approach, on average, than with a transthoracic approach, although it is not clear whether this confers any survival advantage.
- Patients with mid-esophageal tumors (above 32 cm from the incisors) are most easily approached through the chest.
- Patients with end-stage achalasia have an enlarged, tortuous esophagus with enlarged, periesophageal vessels. Transhiatal esophagectomy in this setting is challenging, and transthoracic dissection may be easier.
- Neoadjuvant chemoradiation of gastroesophageal (GE) junction tumors is not a contraindication to this approach as this area is well visualized from the abdomen.
- Patients with poor cardiac function or significant aortic stenosis are best resected with a transthoracic approach in order to avoid perioperative hypotension.
- The transhiatal approach is generally used to reestablish gastrointestinal continuity in patients undergoing cervical exenteration.

Step 2: Preoperative Considerations

- See Chapter 1 for general preoperative considerations.

Step 3: Operative Steps

- The patient is placed in the supine position with both arms to the side. A small transverse bump is placed under the shoulder blades and the head is turned to the right. The abdomen, both anterior chests, and left neck are prepped. A midline laparotomy is performed as described in Chapter 1.

1. Dissection of Esophagus and Cervical Incision

- After mobilization of the gastric conduit as described in Chapter 1, the hiatus is approached. For T2 tumors or smaller, it is acceptable to dissect the crura away from the esophagus. Dissection usually begins on the right and proceeds anteriorly over the left side of the esophagus, which is actually the left limb of the right crus.
- For bulky or T3 tumors, the hiatus should be incised 1 cm away from the tumor and a rim of diaphragm should be incorporated onto the specimen. The phrenic vein, which runs anteriorly, should be ligated. On the right side, the vena cava is located several centimeters away from the esophagus.
- An ultrasonic scalpel may be used to divide all attachments visible from the abdomen. Large arterial branches from the aorta should be clipped. Deaver retractors are useful in gaining exposure. As one proceeds cranially, the Deaver retractors are used to the retract the crus in one direction and a long, large right-angle or Harken #1 clamp can be used to distract the esophagus in the other direction as the assistant uses an ultrasonic scalpel to divide attachments up to the level of the carina.
- At this point an incision is made in the left neck as described in Chapter 1, Tri-Incisional Esophagectomy, with the exception that dissection of the esophagus away from the trachea and recurrent nerves has not already been performed in the chest. (Figure 4-1)
- The sternocleidomastoid and carotid sheath are retracted laterally, and the assistant's finger is used to distract the thyroid and trachea medially. The middle thyroid vein is ligated and divided. The omohyoid is typically divided with cautery.
- The esophagus is identified lying posteriorly to the trachea and anterior to the spine. The nasogastric tube is palpated in the esophagus. The esophagus is sharply separated from the trachea using Metzenbaum scissors. Dissection must be performed immediately on the esophagus in order to avoid the recurrent laryngeal nerves. (Figure 4-2)
- The esophagus is encircled with a Penrose drain, and proximal and distal dissection is performed.
- Circumferential blunt dissection of the esophagus is performed into the thoracic inlet.
- During dissection of the intrathoracic esophagus, the surgeon must be able to see the arterial line tracing. Dissection posterior to the esophagus in the prevertebral plane is generally the easiest and is performed first. Generally the dissection is performed with the palmar aspect of the fingertips against the esophagus. Standing to the right of the patient, the surgeon's right hand is introduced behind the esophagus into the chest. Often the surgeon's left hand is too large to be introduced into the chest from above, and a sponge on a stick is used instead. The right-hand fingertips and sponge stick meet in the mediastinum. Flimsy, intervening tissue is disrupted by a side-to-side rubbing motion, and the two tunnels are united. (Figure 4-3)

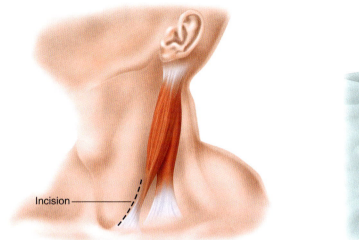

Figure 4-1

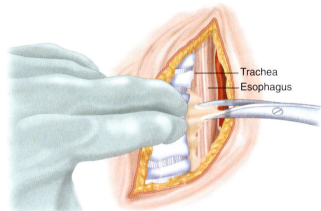

Figure 4-2

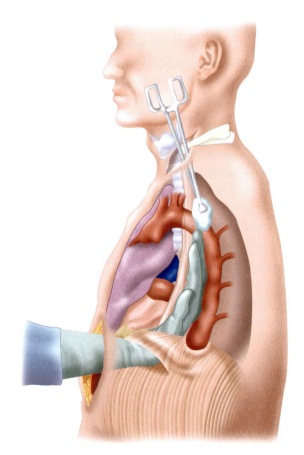

Figure 4-3

- Anterior blunt dissection is next performed from above and below. Extra care is taken near the carina. A gentle side-to-side motion helps distract the esophagus from the membranous trachea. Although a sponge stick can be used for anterior dissection of the esophagus from above, it is reassuring for the surgeon to have both hands in the chest for dissection between the esophagus and trachea. (Figure 4-4)
- After completion of both the anterior and posterior planes, The surgeon's right hand is inserted from below, anterior to the esophagus, until the point of circumferential dissection performed from the neck is reached. The first and second finger surround the esophagus and pin the lateral attachments to the spine. The lateral attachments are avulsed. During this portion of the operation, the recurrent nerves, azygous vein, and branches of the azygous vein are at risk. The surgeon's fingers should stay immediately adjacent to the esophagus. Tough bands to the right of the esophagus near the carina should be assumed to be part of the azygous vein and should be dealt with carefully. (Figure 4-5)
- When dissection is believed to be complete, the upper and lower esophagus are grasped to verify that the entire esophagus is mobile and moves freely. When the esophagus is freely mobile, dissection is complete.

2. Gastric Conduit Pullup and Cervical Anastomosis

- Identical to tri-incisional technique, Chapter 1.

Step 4: Postoperative Care

- The postoperative care is similar to that described in Chapter 1. Any cervical anastomosis places the recurrent nerve at risk, and vocal cord function should be carefully assessed in the first few postoperative days.

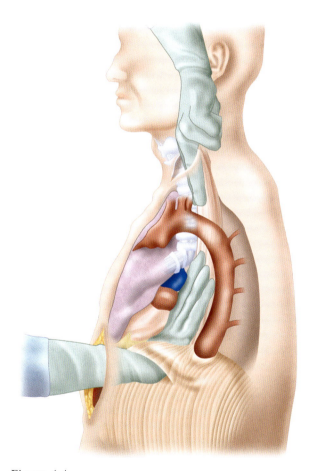

Figure 4-4

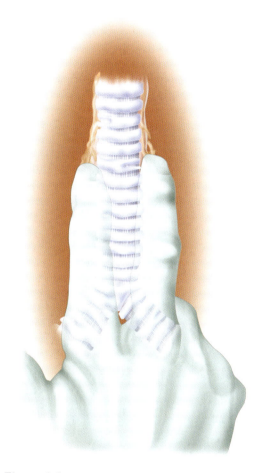

Figure 4-5

Step 5: Pearls and Pitfalls

- If significant difficulty is encountered while dissecting the esophagus bluntly away from the trachea, it is safest to temporarily close the abdominal and neck incisions (with towel clips), place the patient left side down, and dissect the esophagus via right thoracotomy.
- If the membranous aspect of the trachea is entered during transhiatal dissection, the endotracheal tube is gently advanced into the left main bronchus (the surgeon's finger must help with this maneuver as the natural tendency is for the endotracheal tube to go down the right main bronchus) and a right thoracotomy is performed.
- Care must be taken when avulsing lateral attachments to the right of the esophagus near the carina. The azygous vein and its branches are at risk of tearing in this location.
- One must keep track of the pleura on both sides of the dissection. If the pleura is entered intraoperatively, then a chest tube should be placed on that side prior to extubation.

References

1. Chu K, Law S, Wong J, et al. A prospective randomized comparison of transhiatal and transthoracic resection for lower-third esophageal carcinoma. *Am J Surg* 1997; 174:320-324.
2. Goldminc M, Maddern G, LePrise E, et al. Oesophagectomy by a transhiatal approach or thoracotomy: a prospective randomized trial. *Br J Surg* 1993; 80:367-376.
3. Hulscher J, Tijssen J, Lanschot J. Transthoracic versus transhiatal resection for carcinoma of the esophagus: a meta-analysis. *Ann Thor Surg* 2001; 72:306-313.
4. Hulscher J, Van Sandick J, Van Lanschot J. Extended transthoracic resection compared with limited transhiatal resection for adenocarcinoma of the esophagus. *N Engl J Med* 2002; 347:1662-1669.
5. Orringer MB: Esophagectomy without thoracotomy. *J Thorac Cardiovasc Surg* 1978; 76:643.
6. Orringer MB: Technical aids in performing transhiatal esophagectomy without thoracotomy. *Ann Thorac Surg* 1984b; 38:128.
7. Orringer M, Marshall B, Iannettoni M. Transhiatal esophagectomy: clinical experience and refinements. *Ann Surg* 1999; 230:392-403.
8. Rindani R, Martin C, Cox M. Transhiatal versus Ivor-Lewis oesophagectomy: is there a difference? *Aust N Z J Surg* 1999; 69:187-194.

CHAPTER 5

MINIMALLY INVASIVE ESOPHAGECTOMY

Philip A. Linden, MD, FACS, FCCP

Step 1: Surgical Anatomy

- The minimally invasive esophagectomy incorporates either thoracoscopy, laparoscopy, or both, for dissection and reconstruction of the esophagus.
- An EEA anastomosis can be done in the chest, or the conduit may be pulled into the neck for a cervical anastomosis. The equivalent of the tri-incisional approach is described here.
- Thoracoscopic dissection combines the benefits of a thorough lymph node dissection in the chest with less discomfort than seen with open thoracotomy.
- Patients with bulky tumors or tumors of the mid-esophagus (abutting the trachea) are best approached by open thoracotomy.
- Ability to tolerate one-lung anesthesia is essential for adequate visualization during thoracoscopic dissection. Typically this is not a concern even for patients with low FEV_1, unless they are on preoperative oxygen.

Step 2: Preoperative Considerations

- See Chapter 1 for general preoperative considerations.

Step 3: Operative Steps

1. Thoracoscopy

- The patient is placed in the left lateral decubitus position and tilted forward approximately 15 to 20 degrees. Thoracoscopy incisions are performed with the aid of a ring clamp inserted through the skin and used to retract tissues. Muscle layers are carefully cauterized.

- A 10-mm camera port is placed in the midaxillary line in approximately the seventh intercostal space. This first incision should be made under direct vision with blunt entry into the through the pleura to avoid any cautery injury to the underlying lung.
- A 10-mm incision is made in approximately the 4th interspace anterior axillary line.
- A 10-mm incision is made in the 8th or 9th interspace, in line with the tip of the scapula.
- A 5-mm port is placed immediately below the tip of the scapula in approximately the 6th or 7th interspace. (Figures 5-1 and 5-2)
- A #0 Endo Stitch is placed in the central tendon of the diaphragm, and is brought out through a small stab incision in the anterior 8th interspace for inferior retraction of the diaphragm.
- The lung is retracted anteriorly with a fan retractor through the 4th interspace port.
- Most of the dissection is performed with a 5-mm grasper introduced through the port immediately underneath the tip of the scapula, and the ultrasonic shears or 10-mm clipper are inserted through the lower posterior port.
- The inferior pulmonary ligament is divided with cautery.
- The pleura posterior to the esophagus is incised with hook cautery along the length of the esophagus.
- An atraumatic grasper is used to pull the esophagus anteriorly.
- 10-mm clips are used to ligate all arterial branches and lymphatic tissue posterior to the esophagus.
- The ultrasonic scalpel is used anterior to the clips.
- The lower esophagus is distracted posteriorly and the harmonic scalpel is used to dissect the periesophageal tissue away from the pericardium.
- Lifting the esophagus up, the esophagus is encircled with a Penrose drain that may be knotted or stapled.
- The Penrose drain is grasped via the 5-mm port, and ultrasonic scalpel dissection proceeds cranially. Care is taken at the level of the carina and trachea. In general, the insulated side of the ultrasonic shears should be next to trachea when dissecting near the trachea.
- The azygous vein is dissected free with a large right-angle instrument and is divided with an endovascular stapler.
- The vagus nerves at this level are identified and separated from the esophagus.
- The Penrose drain is advanced cranially within the vagus nerves.
- Dissection proceeds to the level of the thoracic inlet, and the knotted Penrose drain is left in the inlet along the spine.
- An additional Penrose drain is placed for retraction, and dissection proceeds toward the diaphragm, which is not opened so as to allow for an adequate pneumoperitoneum during the laparoscopic phase of the dissection.
- A 28F straight chest tube with an additional side hole is placed, the lung is reinflated, and the ports are closed using a 2-0 suture layer on latissimus, 2-0 suture in the subdermal layer, and 3-0 or 4-0 suture in the subcuticular layer.

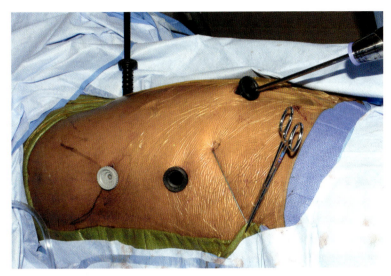

Figure 5-1

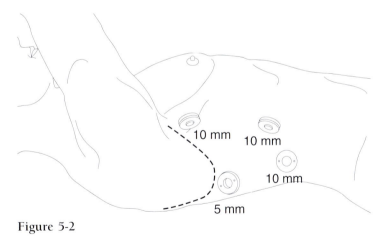

Figure 5-2

2. Laparoscopy

- The patient is placed supine, and the arms are tucked. A padded footboard is placed and the patient is placed in reverse Trendelenburg position. The patient's neck is extended. The surgeon stands to the patient's right.
- Five abdominal ports are used.
- A 12-mm incision is made midway between the midline and right midclavicular line, in the upper abdomen. The anterior fascia, posterior fascia, and peritoneum are opened sharply.
- Additional 5-mm ports are placed laterally on the right (for liver retraction), opposite the 12-mm port on the left, and in higher subcostal positions on the right and left. (Figure 5-3)
- The left lobe of the liver is retracted toward the anterior abdominal wall using either a flexible or a metal retractor.
- A 5-mm, 30-degree camera is placed through the more medial left port (this can be switched with the lateral port position, as needed, during the procedure).
- The ultrasonic scalpel is used to divided the gastrohepatic ligament up to the right crus. The crus is not fully dissected at this point in order to preserve pneumoperitoneum.
- The short gastric vessels are divided using the harmonic scalpel. Repositioning the camera to the left upper quadrant port site facilitates visualization of the highest short gastric vessels.
- Dissection then proceeds inferiorly along the greater curvature, with great care to stay at least 2 cm away from the right gastroepiploic artery.
- The stomach is retracted anteriorly and adhesions are lysed. The left gastric artery pedicle is clamped and divided using a endovascular stapler. Pulsations of the gastroepiploic artery should be visible after clamping, prior to firing of the stapler.
- A Kocher maneuver is performed by retracting all viscera to the patient's left. The ultrasonic shears can be used to carefully grasp and divide the lateral attachments of the duodenum. Additional gentle blunt sweeping dissection can be performed until the duodenum is fully mobilized.
- A pyloroplasty may be performed by placing two retracting 2-0 Endo Stitches, opening the pylorus longitudinally using the harmonic shears, and closing the pyloroplasty transversely using interrupted 2-0 Endo Stitches.
- The nasogastric tube is removed.
- The gastric tube is created by first applying a endovascular staple firing across the right gastric artery to the edge of the lesser curvature of the stomach.
- A thick tissue 4.8-mm stapler is introduced, and the gastric conduit is created with sequential firings. A separate 15-mm port can be introduced into the right upper quadrant for introduction of the stapler.

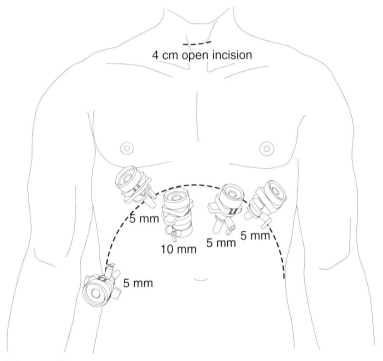

Figure 5-3

- The tip of the gastric tube is attached to the lowest aspects of the esophagogastric specimen using two figure of eight Endo Stitches.
- A point in the jejunum 30 to 40 cm distal to the ligament of Treitz is identified, and a 2-0 Endo Stitch is used to secure the jejunum to the anterior abdominal wall.
- A percutaneous J-tube kit is used to introduce the needle first into the peritoneum just inferior to the stitch and then into the jejunum. The catheter is passed into the jejunum.
- The jejunum is tacked with several circumferential stitches to the abdominal wall, and with an additional stitch 2 cm away from the J-tube in order to prevent torsion.
- Dissection of the crura is performed last. The crural opening is widened.

3. Cervical Incision

- A 6-cm collar-type incision is made from the suprasternal notch extending upward along the anterior border of the sternocleidomastoid muscle.
- The platysma is divided, and blunt dissection down to the spine locates the Penrose drain.
- The esophagus is lifted into the wound.
- The esophagus is divided using a GIA stapler, and the specimen is pulled out through the neck with laparoscopic assistance in guiding the conduit through the hiatus.
- The anastomosis can be performed hand sewn with 3-0 or 4-0 suture, with a 25-mm EEA, or with the technique described in Chapter 1.

Step 4: Postoperative Care

- ◆ The postoperative care is similar to that described in Chapter 1.
- ◆ The small caliber jejunostomy tube inserted via needle clogs easily and should not be used for medication, but for feedings and water only.

Step 5: Pearls and Pitfalls

- ◆ Remove the nasogastric tube prior to stapling the stomach or esophagus.
- ◆ The diaphragmatic hiatus should not be dissected through the chest or abdomen until the end of the laparoscopic dissection so as to preserve the pneumoperitoneum.
- ◆ Lymphatic tissue posterior to the esophagus should be liberally clipped in order to avoid chyle leaks.

References

1. Luiketich J, Alvelo-Rivera M, Buenaventura P, et al. Minimally invasive esophagectomy: outcomes in 222 patients. *Ann Thorac Surg* 2003; 238:486-495.
2. Nguyen N, Follette D, Lemoine P, et al: Minimally invasive Ivor Lewis esophagectomy. *Ann Thorac Surg* 2001; 72:593-596.
3. Swanstrom L, Hansen P. Laparoscopic total esophagectomy. *Arch Surg* 1997; 132:943-949.

CHAPTER 6

NISSEN FUNDOPLICATION

Michael J. Rosen, MD

Step 1: Surgical Anatomy

- Type 1: Sliding hiatal hernia where the gastroesophageal junction herniates within the chest, predisposing to reflux.

Step 2: Preoperative Considerations

- EGD, esophageal motility, and 48-hour Bravo pH
- In special circumstances may order impedance
- Rarely need upper GI unless concern for paraesophageal hernia
- Exclude other causes of symptoms—peptic ulcer disease, achalasia, esophageal dysmotility, and malignancy
- For morbidly obese patients (BMI >40 kg/m^2), consider bariatric surgery

Step 3: Operative Steps

1. **Port Placement and Room Setup** (Figure 6-1AB)

- The room is set up as demonstrated in Figure 6-1. A split leg table approach is preferable. The surgeon stands between the patient's legs. The first assistant stands to the surgeon's right, and the scrub nurse or second assistant stands to the surgeon's left. Dual monitors are placed above the arms. An endoscopy cart is available at the patient's head as well.
- Ports are placed similar to a paraesophageal hernia repair. The initial cutdown port is typically placed one third the distance to the xyphoid process from the umbilicus.
- It is not as critical in a standard Nissen fundoplication to place the ports as high, as an excessive mediastinal dissection is typically not required.

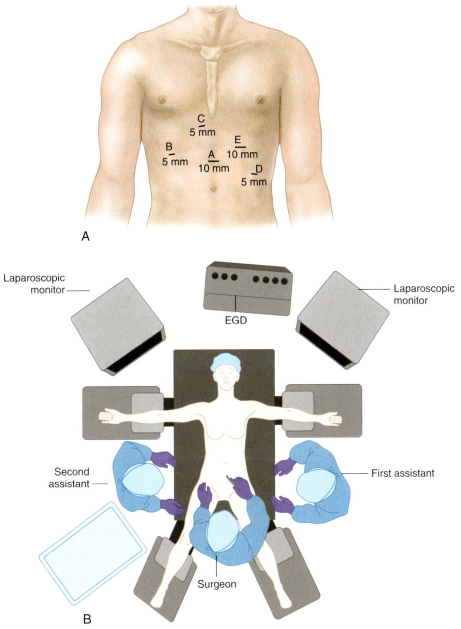

Figure 6-1

2. Dissection at Base of Right Crus (Figure 6-2)

- After division of the gastrohepatic omentum, the right crus is identified.
- It is preferable to begin the hiatal mobilization at the base of the right crus, as this limits the potential for inadvertent esophageal injuries.
- The first assistant grasps the gastroesophageal fat pad and retracts cephalad and to the patient's left. The surgeon grasps the base of the crus as far posteriorly as possible and gently sweeps the phrenoesophageal attachments away. This exposes the decussation of the crural fibers.

3. Dissection of the Right Crus

- After identifying the base of the right crus, the surgeon gently grasps the right crus and sweeps everything medially. In essence this is a crural dissection, and no attempt is made to perform an esophageal dissection at this point. This is an important distinction because early dissection of the esophagus before anatomic structures are clearly identified can result in esophageal injuries.
- The right crus is dissected over the top of the crus until the left vagus is identified, traversing along the anterior esophagus.

4. Division of Short Gastric Vessels

- It is preferable to divide the short gastric vessels prior to exposing the left crus.
- Exposure of the short gastric vessels proceeds in a systematic fashion.
- The surgeon grasps the stomach with the left working port, and the first assistant grasps the gastrosplenic omentum. A common mistake at this point is that the surgeon does not retract the stomach to the patient's right and instead pulls down to the feet. In doing so, the surgeon does not elevate the stomach off the retroperitoneum and makes getting into the appropriate plane more difficult. This is another point at which care must be used to avoid injuring the transverse colon as it can be quite close to the greater curvature of the stomach.
- The dissection plane is approximately 5 to 7 mm off the edge of the stomach. Getting too close to the stomach can result in thermal injuries, and drifting too far away can result in excessive fatty tissue on the stomach or injury to the splenic hilum.
- After entering the lesser sac, the retraction changes. (Figure 6-3) The surgeon places the left hand on the posterior wall of the stomach within the lesser sac and retracts inferiorly and to the left. The first assistant places one side of the grasper in the lesser sac straddling the gastrosplenic omentum. This provides visualization of both the anterior and posterior walls of the stomach prior to division and avoids inadvertent thermal injuries.

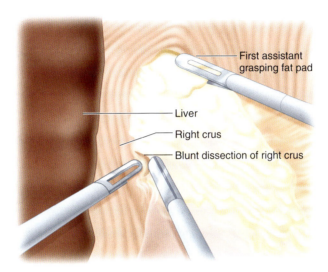

Figure 6-2

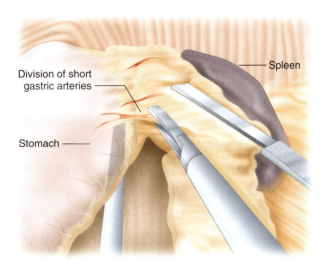

Figure 6-3

- Often the highest short gastric vessel can be challenging to safely expose. To clearly expose this vessel the surgeon now grasps the anterior wall of the stomach and retracts to the patient's right. The first assistant does not need to retract the spleen as the natural splenic attachments provide lateral retraction. Instead the first assistant grasps the posterior wall of the stomach and also retracts to the patient's right.
- If the short gastric pedicle is extremely small, to avoid thermal injury to the stomach or avulsion of the spleen, this vessel can be doubly clipped and divided without the use of an energy source.

5. Division of Second Row of Short Gastrics and Exposure (Figure 6-4)

- There are typically one or two more short gastric vessels located posteromedially. It is important that these are divided to provide a large retroesophageal space for the wrap to sit comfortably. These vessels can come directly off the splenic artery and enter the pancreatic parenchyma, and meticulous hemostasis should be maintained during this portion of the procedure.

6. Passing a Penrose Drain Around the GE Junction

- After division of the short gastrics, the left crus is visualized. A quarter-inch Penrose drain cut at 18 cm is placed in the abdomen and set adjacent to the left crus. The stomach is grasped by the first assistant and retracted to the patient's left. The surgeon then grasps the Penrose drain that is located at the base of the crus that was previously exposed during the initial step of the operation. The Penrose drain is secured tightly around the esophagus with several clips. It is important that the Penrose drain is placed around the esophagus and not the stomach. The Penrose drain is necessary to provide adequate atraumatic retraction of the esophagus for safe dissection. The first assistant grasps the Penrose drain with a locking grasper.

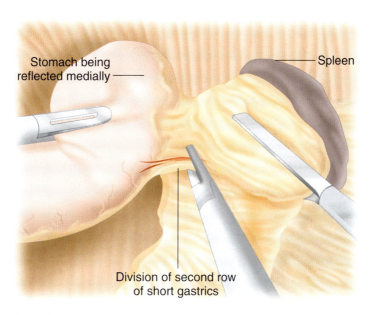

Figure 6-4

7. Complete Left Crus Dissection by Tucking the Penrose Drain Around Fundus

- The first assistant elevates the Penrose drain.
- The surgeon grasps the fundus with the left hand and retracts to the right.
- The first assistant takes the Penrose drain, pulls caudally, tucks the Penrose drain alongside the fundus, and sweeps the entire stomach to the patient's right, exposing the left crus.

8. Mediastinal Mobilization and Esophageal Lengthening

- It is important to gain at least 4 cm of intraabdominal esophagus.
- Retract the Penrose drain inferiorly and bluntly dissect around the esophagus into the mediastinum.
- Typically this is an avascular plane with the exception of a few esophageal aortic branches.
- Take care to carefully identify and preserve the vagus nerves during dissection.
- Avoid stripping the esophagus.

9. Crural Closure (Figure 6-5)

- The crus is typically repaired with 0 braided nylon sutures, pledgets, or mesh when indicated.
- Key to good crural closure is not shredding crura during hiatal dissection and maintaining peritoneal coverage to provide some support.
- Once the hiatus is closed, size the defect with a 56 French bougie. The closure should permit easy passage of a 5-mm-tip suction device.

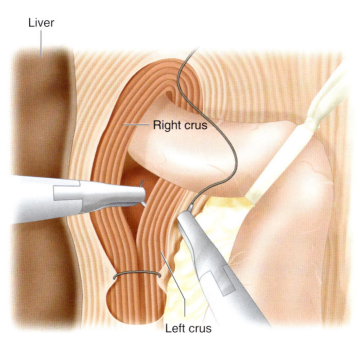

Figure 6-5

10. Construction of Nissen Fundoplication (Figure 6-6ABCD)

- Place an articulating 5-mm endo-go-around to provide angulation to comfortably grasp the posterior fundus.
- The first assistant identifies an area on the posterior fundus to hand to the surgeon.
- The endo-go-around is retracted, bringing the posterior fundus through the retroesophageal window.
- A 56 French bougie is placed down to perform the wrap.
- Perform the shoe shine maneuver. Confirm that the fundus will rest comfortably and is not too tight.
- Suture the anterior wall of the fundus to the esophagus and then to the posterior fundus. Typically three sutures are placed with approximately 2-cm wrap.
- Intraoperative endoscopy can be performed to confirm position of wrap and absence of twisting.

11. Posterior Gastropexy Stitch (Figure 6-7)

- With the completed wrap, the superior posterior portion is sutured to the base of the crural repair to provide intraabdominal fixation.

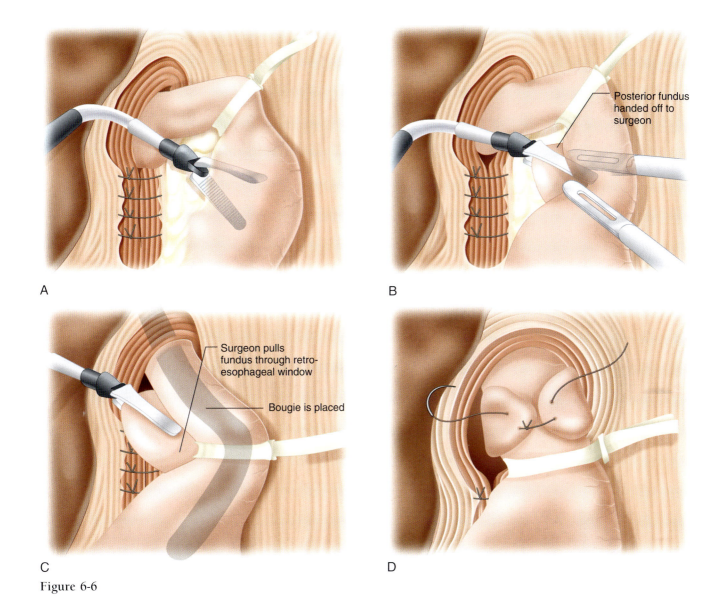

A

B

C

Surgeon pulls
fundus through retro-
esophageal window

Bougie is placed

D

Posterior fundus
handed off to
surgeon

Figure 6-6

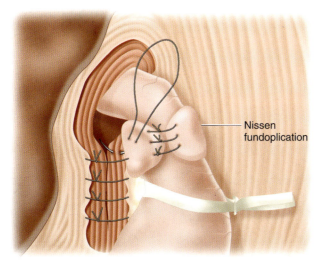

Nissen
fundoplication

Figure 6-7

Step 4: Postoperative Care

- Clear liquids the night of surgery
- No bread, no meat, and no carbonated beverages the next morning; maintained for 2 weeks postoperatively
- Antiemetics given at scheduled times for the first 24 hours, to avoid early retching and early recurrence
- Discharged with prescription for antiemetics
- Swallow only if issues
- Follow up at 2 weeks postoperatively and liberalize diet

Step 5: Pearls and Pitfalls

- Beginning dissection on the phrenoesophageal ligament and inadvertently injuring the esophagus.
- Not dividing the second row of short gastrics and then having an inadequate retroesophageal window for a floppy Nissen.
- Not obtaining adequate intraabdominal esophageal length.
- If one enters the pleura during mediastinal dissection, it is best to make it a large opening to avoid tension pneumothorax. At the end of the procedure, have the anesthesiologist perform the Valsalva maneuver to evacuate CO_2.

- ◆ Closing crura too tightly, predisposing to postoperative dysphagia. This can be difficult to treat.
- ◆ Constructing an inappropriately configured wrap, either twisting or bringing the body to the fundus.
- ◆ It is important that patients understand the incidence of transient postoperative dysphagia and gas bloating symptoms.

References

1. Oelschlager BK, Quiroga E, Parra JD, et al. Long-term outcomes after laparoscopic antireflux surgery. *Am J Gastroenterol* 2008; 103:280-287; quiz 288.
2. Robertson AG, Dunn LJ, Shenfine J, et al. Randomized clinical trial of laparoscopic total (Nissen) versus posterior partial (Toupet) fundoplication for gastro-oesophageal reflux disease based on preoperative oesophageal manometry. *Br J Surg* 2008; 95: 57-63.
3. Salminen PT, Hiekkanen HI, Rantala AP, et al. Comparison of long-term outcome of laparoscopic and conventional nissen fundoplication: a prospective randomized study with an 11-year follow-up. *Ann Surg* 2007; 246: 201-206.

CHAPTER 7

PARAESOPHAGEAL HERNIA REPAIR

Michael J. Rosen, MD

Step 1: Surgical Anatomy

1. **Types of Paraesophageal Hernias** (Figure 7-1ABCDE)

   - Type 1: Sliding hiatal hernia in which the gastroesophageal junction moves cephalad, predisposing to gastroesophageal reflux.
   - Type 2: Rare hernias in which the gastroesophageal junction remains in its normal anatomic position, and the fundus herniates alongside it into the chest.
   - Type 3: Classic paraesophageal hernia, in which there are a combination of a type 1 and 2 hernias. Both the gastroesophageal junction and the fundus herniate into the chest. These hernias can be associated with organoaxial rotation predisposing to incarceration.
   - Type 4: Involves another intraabdominal organ within the hernia sac.

2. **Anatomy of hernia sac** (Figure 7-2)

   - This is a cross-sectional image of the hernia sac demonstrating both an anterior and posterior component. The hernia sac is bisected by the stomach and its gastrohepatic and gastrosplenic ligaments. Both the anterior and posterior sac must be reduced from the mediastinum to complete an adequate paraesophageal hernia repair.

Hiatal Hernia: Types

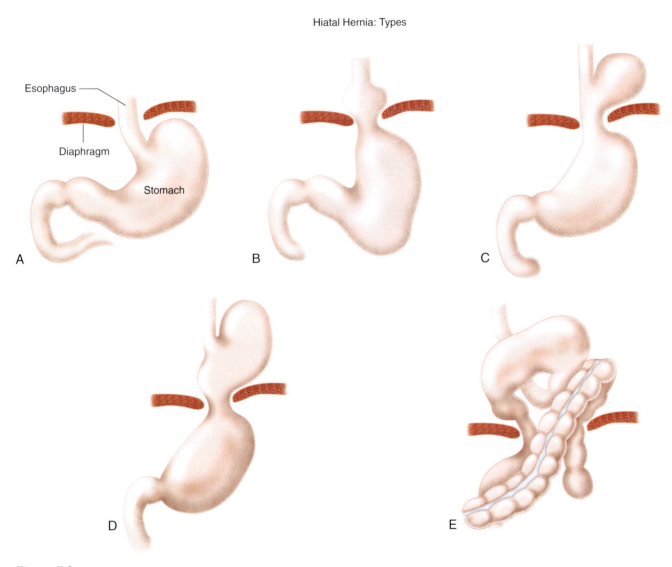

Figure 7-1

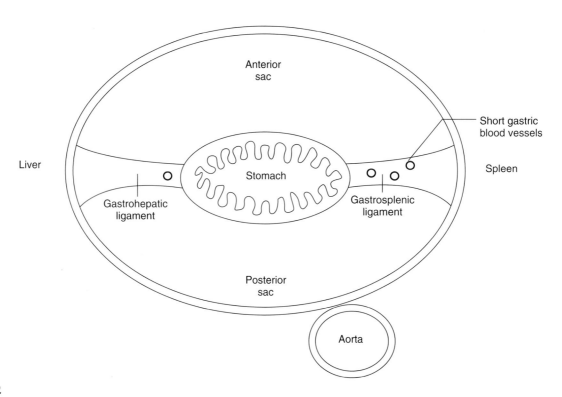

Figure 7-2

Step 2: Preoperative Considerations

1. Preoperative Work-Up

- Appropriate cardiac and pulmonary clearance as indicated.
- Video barium swallow: Provides anatomic assessment and classification of type of hiatal hernia, paraesophageal component, and esophageal length. The video swallow can also assess esophageal function.
- Upper endoscopy: Rules out intrinsic esophageal lesions and allows assessment of esophageal length.
- Esophageal motility: This is not routinely ordered as it can be difficult to accurately place a catheter with anatomic distortion.
- 24-hour pH study: This is not routinely ordered.

Step 3: Operative Steps

1. Port Placement

- Port A: Initial access is gained with an open cut-down technique approximately one third of the distance from the umbilicus to the xiphoid process. It is important that this port is placed no more than 14 cm from the xiphoid process or the camera will not be able to reach high enough to perform an adequate mediastinal dissection.
- Port B: 5-mm liver retractor. This port should be placed fairly cephalad to avoid interfering with the surgeon's left operative port.
- Port C: With the liver retractor in place and the left lateral segment of the liver elevated, the next 5-mm port is placed. It is preferable to place this to the patient's left of the falciform ligament to avoid interference during instrument exchanges. It should be placed just inferior to the left lateral segment of the liver.
- Port D: 5-mm first assistant port. This should be placed as far lateral as possible, just inferior to the costal margin.
- Port E: 10-mm surgeon's right-hand working port. This port is placed at least a hand's breadth away from port C to provide adequate separation, to allow suturing. In patients with a narrow costal margin this should be placed closer to port D to avoid crowding of the surgeon's two working instruments.

2. Initial Dissection

- A gentle manual reduction of the hernia contents is initially attempted. The main purpose of this maneuver is to allow some pneumoperitoneum to enter the hernia sac to make dissection easier. No attempt should be made to dissect adhesions within the hernia sac, as the true dissection plane is outside of the hernia sac.
- The first assistant grasps the stomach and retracts to the patient's left, and the surgeon divides the gastrohepatic ligament. This dissection should be carried cephalad until the right crus is identified. Care should be taken to avoid injuring an accessory left hepatic artery (see Pearls and Pitfalls).

3. Initial Hernia Sac Dissection (Figure 7-3)

- This is one of the most critical steps in the procedure. It is important to identify the proper dissection plane to avoid excessive bleeding and damage to major mediastinal structures. It is preferable to begin this dissection at approximately the 11 o'clock position. Typically this is the insertion point of the gastrohepatic ligament into the right crus, and it tends to be the thickest part of the phrenoesophageal ligament. Additionally it is important to begin this plane approximately 3 to 4 mm on the abdominal side of the crus. If the dissection is started further on the abdominal side, the peritoneal covering of the crus is often disrupted, making eventual suture repair very difficult during later steps in the procedure. If the dissection is begun too far in the mediastinum, the hernia sac retracts into the mediastinum and can be difficult to control.
- The first assistant grasps the peritoneal edge and the surgeon uses the harmonic to divide the peritoneal coverage of the crus. This plane is all the way down to the muscular fibers of the crus.

4. Mediastinal Sac Dissection

- Once the appropriate plane is entered, the first assistant grasps the hernia sac and retracts caudally. The majority of the hernia sac dissection should be performed bluntly. If the surgeon is in the correct plane few to no blood vessels should be encountered.
- This maneuver is performed by placing the two tips of the surgeon's instruments together and pushing away from each other in either an up-and-down or side-to-side motion. This dissection is continued from the 11 o'clock position over the top of the crus to the 3 o'clock position.
- The hernia sac should be reduced out of the left chest. As the sac is reduced out of the left chest the aorta will come into view.
- At this point, do not perform extensive dissection at the apex of the hernia sac as this can result in inadvertent injury of the esophagus.

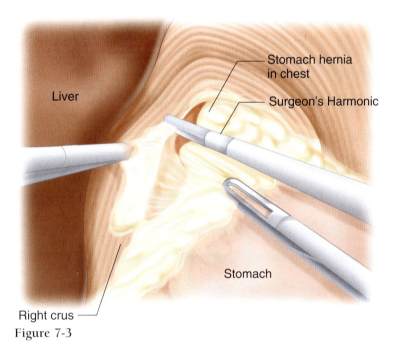

Liver

Stomach hernia
in chest

Surgeon's Harmonic

Stomach

Right crus

Figure 7-3

5. Right Crural Dissection

◆ With the first assistant grasping the hernia sac, the surgeon reduces the sac from the right chest. This begins the posterior hernia sac dissection. Again, care should be taken to avoid destroying these crural fibers during this part of the dissection. The right crus should be dissected to its base until the fibers of the left crus are encountered. At this point only the lower part of the left crus remains to be dissected. This can be a difficult area to expose and it is preferable to divide the short gastric vessels to enhance exposure.

6. Divide Short Gastrics

◆ The short gastric dissection is begun at the mid body of the stomach. Once the short gastrics are divided, there is typically a second row of short gastrics that must be divided posteriorly. Once this retroesophageal window is created a Penrose drain is secured around the esophagus.

7. Exposure of the Left Crus with Penrose Drain. (Figure 7-4AB)

◆ Adequate exposure of the left crus with a floppy fundus can be challenging.
◆ With the first assistant elevating the Penrose drain, the surgeon grasps the apex of the fundus with his or her left hand and retracts it to the patient's right. The first assistant then uses the Penrose drain as a retractor to tuck the fundus, and bluntly pushes the Penrose drain to the patient's right to expose the base of the left crus.
◆ If excessive gastrosplenic omental fat gets in the way, see Pearls and Pitfalls.

8. Mediastinal Esophageal Mobilization (Figure 7-5)

◆ Appropriate mediastinal esophageal mobilization is critical to obtain adequate intraabdominal esophageal length and provide scarring of this space to reduce recurrence rates.
◆ This space is largely avascular, with the exception of a few esophageal vessels coming directly off the aorta. These can typically be divided with the harmonic. If bleeding is encountered, typically a 3 × 3-inch sponge can be used to provide hemostasis, or alternatively small clips may be used.
◆ Care should be taken to avoid injuring or dividing the vagus nerves.
◆ This dissection should be carried high into the mediastinum. With adequate dissection, shortened esophagus is very uncommon.

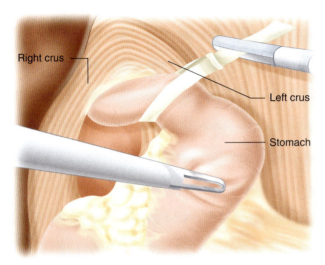

Right crus

Left crus

Stomach

A

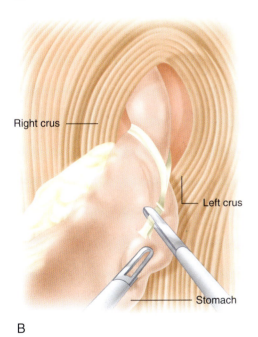

Right crus

Left crus

Stomach

B

Figure 7-4

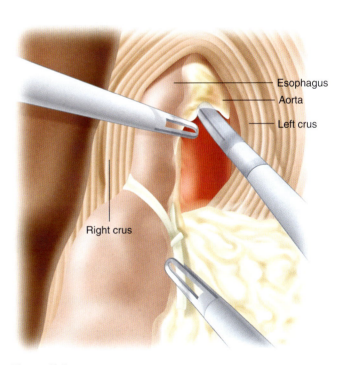

Esophagus

Aorta

Left crus

Right crus

Figure 7-5

9. Crural Closure (Figure 7-6AB)

◆ There are multiple methods available to close the crura.
◆ Primary repair with a permanent suture is preferable.
◆ If excessive tension is encountered, pledgets may be used.
◆ In situations where the crural fibers are significantly attenuated, an onlay of biologic mesh can be onlayed.
◆ In the rare event that the crus simply can not be brought together, a soft piece of ePTFE mesh can be placed as a bridge repair.

10. Fundoplication

◆ Most patients will have some symptoms of reflux after the hiatal dissection necessary to complete a paraesophageal hernia repair.
◆ One of the main advantages of an antireflux procedure is to provide further intraabdominal fixation of the stomach.
◆ Either a Nissen or a Toupet fundoplication is acceptable in this situation (see Chapter 8, Heller Myotomy).
◆ After performing the fundoplication, a posterior gastropexy suture is placed. This secures the posterior aspect of the wrap to the crural repair.
◆ If adequate esophageal length cannot be obtained to perform a fundoplication, instead of performing esophageal lengthening procedures, the anterior gastropexy described in this chapter may be performed.

11. Anterior Gastropexy (Figure 7-7)

◆ To provide further intraabdominal gastric fixation, two 0 Prolene sutures can be placed into the anterior gastric wall. These sutures should be placed along the lesser curvature of the stomach and used to place the stomach on mild caudal traction. In doing so, the angle of His is recreated, providing some antireflux effect.
◆ Once the sutures are placed in the anterior wall of the stomach the needle is removed. Using a suture passer similar to a laparoscopic ventral hernia repair, through a single skin incision, the needle passer retrieves each of the tails through separate fascial punctures. The suture is then secured in a subcutaneous position.

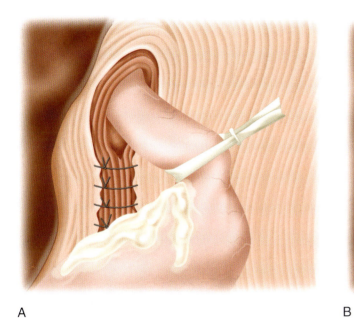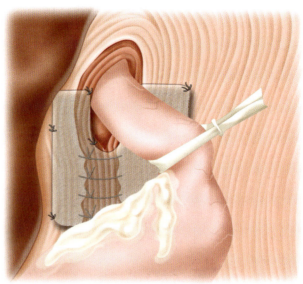

A   B

Figure 7-6

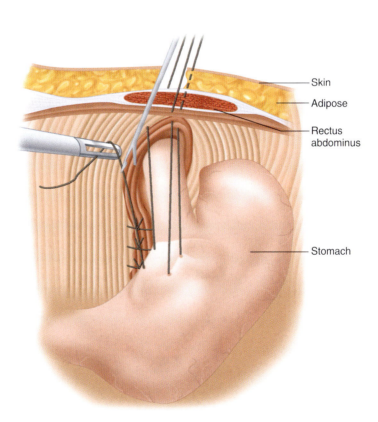

Figure 7-7

Step 4: Postoperative Care

- NPO till AM
- Gastrograffin swallow in AM
- No bread, no meat, and no carbonated beverages for 2 weeks
- Antiemetics around the clock for 24 hours
- Discharged with prescription or antinausea medicine
- Seen 2 weeks postoperatively and diet liberalized

Step 5: Pearls and Pitfalls

- It is imperative that ports are placed in a cephalad position. If ports are placed too low, the instruments will not reach into the chest.
- Accessory left hepatic artery: Encountering this vessel can make dissection difficult. Typically this can be clipped and divided with little consequence. In the event of encountering a substantial left hepatic vessel and perhaps a replaced left hepatic, a clip can be placed on the vessel during the initial dissection. The hepatic vessel is not divided at this point. The remainder of the dissection is continued, and after several minutes the liver is assessed for signs of ischemia. If the liver appears ischemic, more length can be achieved from the left hepatic by dissecting it down to its insertion in either the left gastric or celiac axis.
- During sac dissection, try and maintain peritoneal coverage over the crus. If the crural fibers are destroyed during this part of the dissection, the eventual repair will be difficult.
- If excessive fat from the gastrosplenic ligament obscures exposure of the left crus, one can place an endoloop around the omentum and retrieve the tail with a suture passer, and place it under traction externally by clipping to the skin, to improve exposure without losing a surgical instrument.

- The use of esophageal lengthening procedures is controversial in paraesophageal hernia repairs. Adequate mediastinal esophageal mobilization can avoid this problem. In the rare circumstance where a shortened esophagus is encountered, it is typically preferable to avoid lengthening procedures. As mentioned previously these procedures are typically performed in elderly patients to avoid life-threatening complications of organoaxial rotation. If a small sliding hiatal hernia is left, this can typically be controlled well with antireflux medication. This avoids placing of staple lines near the gastroesophageal junction in this patient population, which is necessary when performing a lengthening procedure.
- With the stomach in the chest for many years and the excessive dissection around the vagus nerve, postoperative delayed gastric emptying is common in this patient population. While this is typically self-limiting, postoperative retching can result in early recurrence. Options for managing this problem include Botox injection of the pylorus, medical therapy, or gastrostomy tube placement.

References

1. Hashemi M, Peters JH, DeMeester TR, et al. Laparoscopic repair of large type III hiatal hernia: objective followup reveals high recurrence rate. *J Am Coll Surg* 2000; 190:553-60; discussion 560-561.
2. Pierre AF, Luketich JD, Fernando HC, et al. Results of laparoscopic repair of giant paraesophageal hernias: 200 consecutive patients. *Ann Thorac Surg* 2002; 74:1909-15; discussion 1915-1916.
3. Ponsky J, Rosen M, Fanning A, et al. Anterior gastropexy may reduce the recurrence rate after laparoscopic paraesophageal hernia repair. *Surg Endosc* 2003; 17:1036-1041.
4. Schauer PR, Ikramuddin S, McLaughlin RH, et al. Comparison of laparoscopic versus open repair of paraesophageal hernia. *Am J Surg* 1998; 176:659-665.
5. Stylopoulos N, Rattner DW. Paraesophageal hernia: when to operate? *Adv Surg* 2003; 37:213-229.

CHAPTER 8

HELLER MYOTOMY

Michael J. Rosen, MD

Step 1: Surgical Anatomy

- ◆ Esophageal muscular layers: outer longitudinal, middle circular, inner layer mucosa
- ◆ Gastric muscular layers: outer longitudinal, middle circular, inner oblique, mucosa
- ◆ Cause of achalasia: destruction of esophageal myoenteric plexus

Step 2: Preoperative Considerations

- ◆ Typical presentation includes progressive dysphagia to solids and liquids.
- ◆ Nonoperative therapy:
  - ▲ Medical treatment: nitrates, calcium channel blockers
  - ▲ Endoscopic therapy
    Pneumatic dilatation
    Botulinum toxin injection
- ◆ Preoperative evaluation:
  - ▲ Endoscopy: rules out pseudoachalasia
  - ▲ Esophageal motility studies: aperistaltic esophageal body, failure of relaxation of gastro-esophageal junction with swallowing
    Upper GI study: classic "birdsbeak"
    24-hour pH: inaccurate

Step 3: Operative Steps

1. Port Positioning

- ◆ This is similar to Nissen fundoplication.

2. Hiatal Dissection

- It is preferable to perform a circumferential esophageal dissection to perform a Heller myotomy, similar to a Nissen (see Chapter 6). This allows placement of a Penrose drain around the gastroesophageal junction to provide downward traction during the proximal extension of the myotomy. We also routinely divide the short gastric vessels during this dissection as we feel it is necessary when performing a Toupet or Dor fundoplication at the end of the procedure.

3. Identification of Anterior Vagal Nerves (Figure 8-1)

- Identification of the vagal nerve prior to performing the myotomy is important to avoid inadvertent transection. After identifying the vagal nerve it is encircled with a 0-silk suture. The two tails are clipped together, and the vagus nerve is bluntly dissected off the esophagus for the length of the myotomy. During the myotomy, the surgeon can control the path of the vagus nerve by grasping and retracting the prior placed sutures. If a large esophageal fat pad is encountered, it should be resected.

4. Preinjection of Dilute Epinephrine (Figure 8-2)

- In order to avoid excessive bleeding during the myotomy, a dilute solution of epinephrine can be injected into the esophageal wall with a long, 22-gauge spinal needle. The surgeon should stabilize the tip of this needle with a grasper, insure injection into the muscular plane, and avoid intraluminal injection.

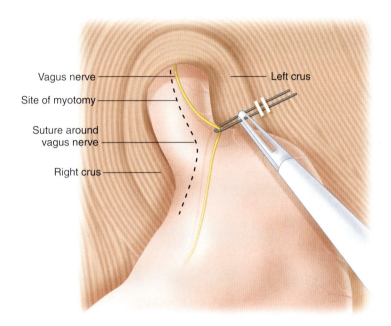

Vagus nerve

Left crus

Site of myotomy

Suture around
vagus nerve

Right crus

Figure 8-1

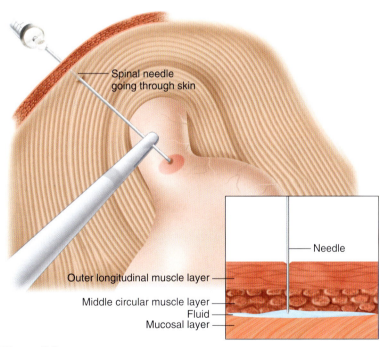

Spinal needle
going through skin

Needle

Outer longitudinal muscle layer

Middle circular muscle layer

Fluid

Mucosal layer

Figure 8-2

5. **Myotomy** (Figure 8-3)

◆ The myotomy is begun approximately 2 cm above the gastroesophageal junction. Initially the longitudinal layers are separated, then the circular muscles are divided with the hook cautery. The use of electrical sources is minimized for this dissection. The hook is typically at very low settings of 10 volts. If bleeding is encountered, avoid excessive cautery and use pressure instead.
◆ The myotomy is extended at least 6 to 7 cm proximal along the esophagus. (Figure 8-4)
◆ The myotomy is then extended at least 3 cm onto the gastric wall. (Figure 8-5)

6. **Intraoperative Endoscopy**

◆ An EGD is performed to confirm the completeness of the myotomy as the scope should easily pass into the stomach. It also is performed to rule out an intraoperative perforation.

7. **Toupet Fundoplication** (Figure 8-6)

◆ If one performs a circumferential esophageal mobilization, a posterior 270-degree fundoplication can be performed. Typically three sutures are placed on each side, with the fundus secured to each edge of the cut myotomy. This may provide a slight advantage as an antireflux procedure but can cause anterior angulation of the esophagus and potentially more dysphagia.

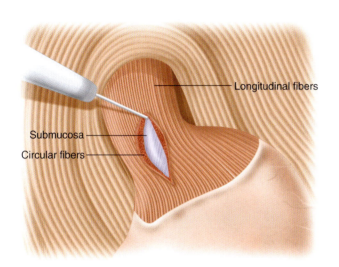

Longitudinal fibers

Submucosa

Circular fibers

Figure 8-3

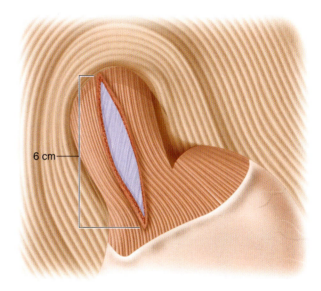

6 cm

Figure 8-4

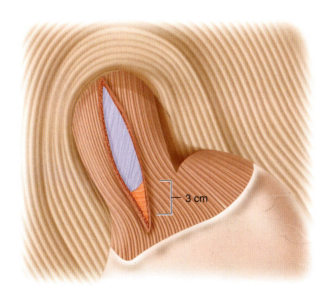

3 cm

Figure 8-5

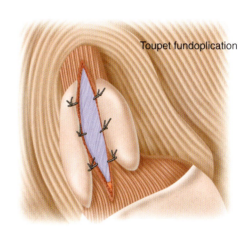

Toupet fundoplication

Figure 8-6

8. Dor Fundoplication (Figure 8-7AB)

- Figure 7A: The apex of the fundus is grasped and retracted cephalad alongside the myotomy. It is important to recreate the acute angle of the angle of His. This likely provides the antireflux effect of the Dor fundoplication. Several sutures are placed to secure the fundus to the cut edge of the myotomy.
- Figure 7B: The fundus is then wrapped over the myotomy and secured to the right crus with at least three sutures.

Step 4: Postoperative Care

- NPO till AM
- Swallow in AM
- Soft diet, home after lunch

Step 5: Pearls and Pitfalls

- If bleeding is encountered during the myotomy, avoid using excessive cautery to prevent a potential mucosal injury resulting in a delayed esophageal perforation. A 1 × 1 cm section of surgicele soaked in the dilute epinephrine can be placed on the small bleeding vessels and dissection performed elsewhere.
- If the esophagus is perforated during the myotomy, the hole can be closed with an absorbable suture. If it is a small perforation, continue the myotomy and perform a Dor fundoplication to buttress the repair. If it is a large perforation, close all layers of the esophagus over the perforation and perform the myotomy on the posterolateral wall of the esophagus.
- If patients have had prior pneumatic dilatation or botulinum injection treatments, the myotomy plane can be severely scarred and difficult to maintain.

References

1. Kostic S, Kjellin A, Ruth M, et al. Pneumatic dilatation or laparoscopic cardiomyotomy in the management of newly diagnosed idiopathic achalasia. Results of a randomized controlled trial. *World J Surg* 2007; 31:470-478.
2. Patti MG, Fisichella PM, Perretta S, et al. Impact of minimally invasive surgery on the treatment of esophageal achalasia: a decade of change. *J Am Coll Surg* 2003; 196:698-703; discussion 703-705.
3. Richards WO, Torquati A, Holzman MD, et al. Heller myotomy versus Heller myotomy with Dor fundoplication for achalasia: a prospective randomized double-blind clinical trial. *Ann Surg* 2004; 240:405-412; discussion 412-415.
4. Rossetti G, Brusciano L, Amato G, et al. A total fundoplication is not an obstacle to esophageal emptying after Heller myotomy for achalasia: results of a long-term follow up. *Ann Surg* 2005; 241:614-621.
5. Sharp KW, Khaitan L, Scholz S, et al. 100 consecutive minimally invasive Heller myotomies: lessons learned. *Ann Surg* 2002; 235:631-638; discussion 638-9.

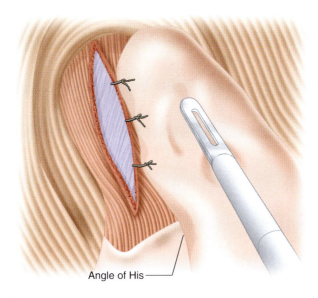

Angle of His

A

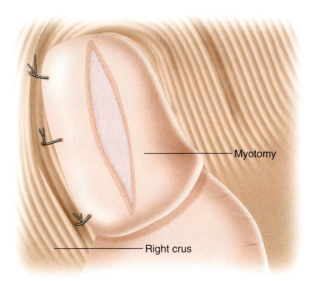

Myotomy

Right crus

B

Figure 8-7

CHAPTER 9

TRUNCAL VAGOTOMY

Alfredo M. Carbonell, DO, FACS, FACOS

Step 1: Surgical Anatomy

- The anterior or left vagus nerve is a thick, visible structure which lies just right of the midline along the anterior surface of the intraabdominal esophagus. (Figures 9-1 and 9-2)
- The posterior, or right vagus nerve, is thinner and lies to the right of the esophagus, closer to the aorta than the esophagus. (Figures 9-1 and 9-2) Palpation of a thin cord posterior to the esophagus will typically reveal its location.
- Truncal vagotomy requires skeletonization of the anterior and posterior vagus nerve trunks with complete transection.

Step 2: Preoperative Considerations

- When performed properly, a complete truncal vagotomy results in denervation of the stomach, liver, gallbladder, pancreas, small intestine, and proximal large intestine.
- As the gastric antral pump is denervated, a concomitant gastric drainage (pyloroplasty, gastro-jejunostomy) or resective (antrectomy) procedure is recommended.

Step 3: Operative Steps

1. Positioning and Incision

- The patient is positioned supine with both arms extended. A footboard is attached to the bed to support the patient.
- A midline incision allows for sufficient visualization of the upper stomach and esophagus.

72

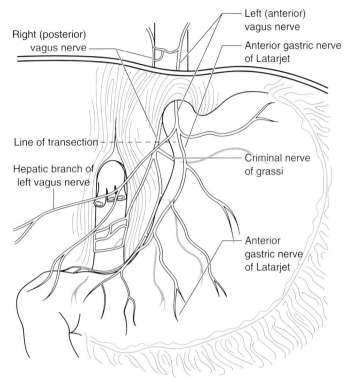

Left (anterior)
vagus nerve

Right (posterior)
vagus nerve

Anterior gastric nerve
of Latarjet

Line of transection

Criminal nerve
of grassi

Hepatic branch of
left vagus nerve

Anterior
gastric nerve
of Latarjet

Figure 9-1

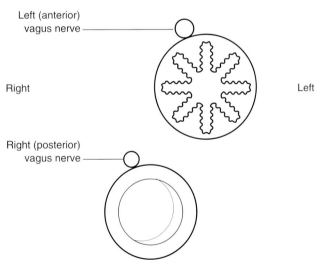

Left (anterior)
vagus nerve

Right

Left

Right (posterior)
vagus nerve

Figure 9-2

♦ An abdominal wall retractor is placed for cephalad retraction. A sweetheart retractor attachment is placed in the midline to gently retract the junction of the esophagus and diaphragm. The patient is placed in steep reverse Trendelenburg position.
♦ An orogastric tube is advanced into the proximal stomach; this helps serve as a guide for palpation of the esophagus.
♦ The operating surgeon stands to the patient's right.

2. Dissection

♦ The gastrophrenic ligament is divided and the dissection carried over the anterior portion of the phrenoesophageal ligament toward the gastrohepatic ligament. (Figure 9-3)
♦ The surgeon's right index finger is passed posterior-superior into the mediastinum to encircle the esophagus. The dissection should be directed onto the aorta as the posterior vagus nerve may be adherent to the aorta.
♦ The index finger is advanced and brought out adjacent to the right crus. The posterior vagus nerve can be palpated as a taut band on the posterior aspect of the esophagus. (Figure 9-4)
♦ With the surgeon's right hand in place, the assistant skeletonizes an approximate 6-cm length of vagus nerve into the mediastinum. The nerve is then clipped proximally and distally and a 2-cm section is resected and sent fresh to pathology for frozen section. (Figure 9-5)
♦ Anterior vagal dissection proceeds by isolating and transecting small branches of the anterior vagus nerve along a 6-cm length of the nerve. Clips are placed proximally and distally, and a 2-cm section of the nerve is sent for frozen section. (Figure 9-6)

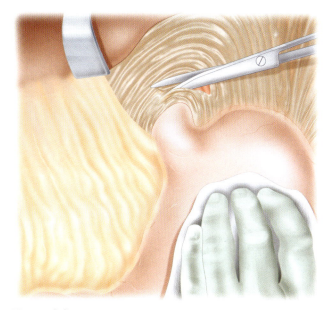

Figure 9-3

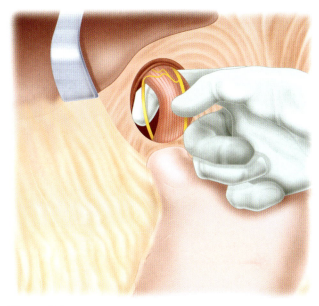

Figure 9-4

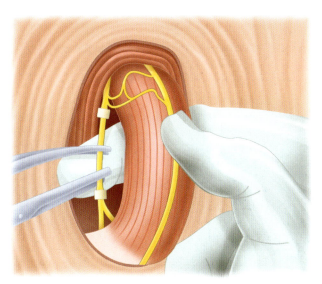

Figure 9-5

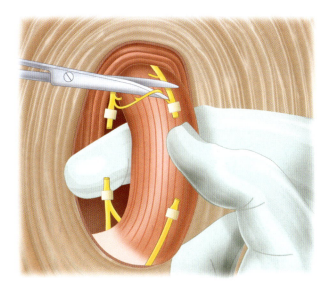

Figure 9-6

Step 4: Postoperative Care

- ◆ The patient may be started on a diet after surgery and advanced as tolerated.

Step 5: Pearls and Pitfalls

- ◆ Complete skeletonization of the vagus nerves ensures the transection of small intervening nerve branches. Failure to transect these small branches may result in an incomplete vagotomy.
- ◆ The "criminal nerve" of Grassi is the first gastric branch of the posterior vagus nerve. This nerve may branch proximal or distal to the celiac division of the posterior vagus nerve. The importance of skeletonizing an adequate length of the posterior vagus nerve into the mediastinum cannot be overemphasized, as failure to transect the nerve of Grassi proximal to its origin will result in an incomplete vagotomy.

References

1. Dragstedt LR, 2nd, Lulu DJ. Truncal vagotomy and pyloroplasty. Critical evaluation of one hundred cases. *Am J Surg* 1974; 128(3):344-346.
2. Foster JH. Pyloroplasty, vagotomy, and suture ligation for bleeding duodenal ulcer. In: Nyhus LM, Baker RJ, Fischer JE, eds. *Mastery of surgery*. Vol. 1. Boston: Little, Brown and Company; 1997.
3. Skandalakis JE, Skandalakis PN, Skandalakis LJ. *Surgical anatomy and technique*. New York: Springer-Verlag; 1995.
4. Skandalakis LJ, Donahue PE, Skandalakis JE. The vagus nerve and its vagaries. *Surg Clin North Am* 1993; 73(4):769-784.

SELECTIVE VAGOTOMY

Alfredo M. Carbonell, DO, FACS, FACOS

Step 1: Surgical Anatomy

- Selective vagotomy entails transection of both the descending branch of the anterior vagus nerve (anterior nerve of Latarjet) distal to the hepatic branches, and the descending branch of the posterior vagus (posterior nerve of Latarjet) distal to the celiac branches. (Figure 10-1)

Step 2: Preoperative Considerations

- Similar to truncal vagotomy, selective vagotomy completely denervates the stomach and requires a concomitant gastric drainage or resective procedure.
- The solitary pyloric branch of the hepatic division of the anterior vagus nerve and the celiac branches of the posterior vagus nerve are undisturbed, preserving the innervation to the biliary tract, small bowel, and proximal large bowel.
- Selective vagotomy is the least performed of all the vagotomy subtypes likely due to the difficulty in identifying the celiac branch of the posterior vagus nerve.

Step 3: Operative Steps

1. Positioning and Incision

- The patient is positioned supine with both arms extended. A footboard is attached to the bed to support the patient.
- A midline incision allows for sufficient visualization of the upper stomach and esophagus.
- An abdominal wall retractor is placed for cephalad retraction. A sweetheart retractor attachment is placed in the midline to gently retract the junction of the esophagus and diaphragm. The patient is placed in steep reverse Trendelenburg position.
- An orogastric tube is advanced into the proximal stomach and helps serve as a guide for palpation of the esophagus.
- The operating surgeon stands to the patient's right.

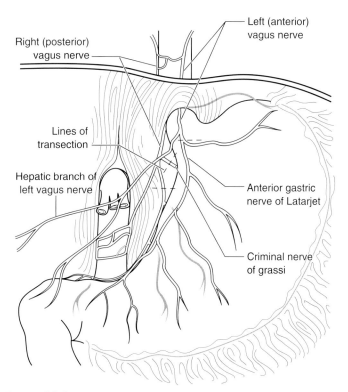

Figure 10-1

2. Dissection

- The gastrophrenic ligament is divided and the dissection carried over the anterior portion of the phrenoesophageal ligament towards to the gastrohepatic ligament. (Figure 10-2)
- Mobilization is carried out similar to the truncal vagotomy. The surgeon's right index finger is passed posterior-superior into the mediastinum to encircle the esophagus.
- The index finger is advanced and brought out adjacent to the right crus. The posterior vagus nerve can be palpated as a taut band on the posterior aspect of the esophagus. (Figure 10-3)
- With the surgeon's right hand in place, the assistant aids in skeletonizing the posterior vagus nerve above and below the level of the celiac branch. This ensures complete division of the first gastric branch of the posterior vagus (nerve of Grassi), which will course to the patient's left. The main posterior gastric division (posterior nerve of Latarjet) is then clipped and transected distal to the celiac branch, which will course to the patient's right. (Figure 10-4)
- The anterior vagus nerve and its first hepatic branch coursing to the patient's right are identified. The anterior nerve of Laterjet is isolated distal to the hepatic division, then clipped and divided. (Figure 10-5)

Step 4: Postoperative Care

- The patient may be started on a diet after surgery and advanced as tolerated.

Step 5: Pearls and Pitfalls

- There is great anatomic variability of the anterior vagus nerve and its branches within the abdomen. If the proximal hepatic division is not identified coursing to the patient's right, the anterior nerve of Latarjet is traced inferiorly along the lesser curve until the hepatic division can be seen branching.
- It is possible for there to be a double anterior nerve of Latarjet or none at all. In the latter case, the gastric branches come off the hepatic division, and should be transected proximal to their entry into the lesser curve of the stomach.
- Although there is anatomic variability of the posterior vagus nerve as well, the one constant is the celiac division will be the largest of the vagal divisions. It is always single, and leads directly to the celiac plexus, following the left gastric artery or right crus of the diaphragm.

References

1. Johnston D, Blackett RL. A new look at selective vagotomies. *Am J Surg* 1988; 156(5):416-427.
2. Sawyers JL. Selective vagotomy and pyloroplasty. In: Nyhus LM, Baker RJ, Fischer JE, eds. *Mastery of surgery.* Vol. 1. Boston: Little, Brown and Company; 1997.
3. Skandalakis JE, Skandalakis PN, Skandalakis LJ. *Stomach. Surgical anatomy and technique.* New York: Springer-Verlag; 1995.
4. Skandalakis LJ, Donahue PE, Skandalakis JE. The vagus nerve and its vagaries. *Surg Clin North Am* 1993; 73(4):769-784.

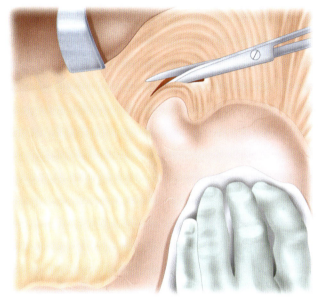

Figure 10-2

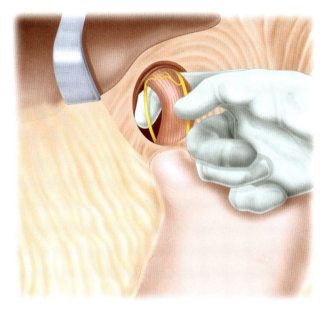

Figure 10-3

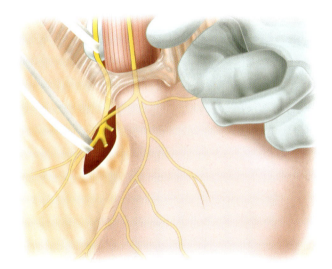

Figure 10-4

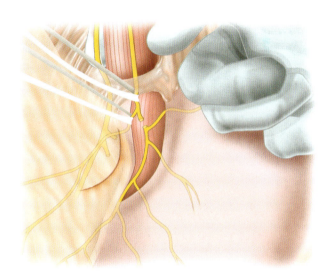

Figure 10-5

CHAPTER 11

HIGHLY SELECTIVE VAGOTOMY

Alfredo M. Carbonell, DO, FACS, FACOS

Step 1: Surgical Anatomy

- After giving off the hepatic branch, the anterior nerve of Latarjet courses inferiorly, within the anterior leaflet of the gastrohepatic ligament, medial to the lesser curve.
- Similarly, after giving off the celiac branch, the posterior nerve of Latarjet courses inferiorly, within the posterior leaflet of the gastrohepatic ligament, medial to the lesser curve.
- Both nerves of Latarjet terminate with branches to the antrum and pylorus. Although classically described resembling a crow's foot configuration, this fan-like configuration of nerves is inconsistent.
- Highly selective vagotomy (HSV) or parietal cell vagotomy entails transection of the proximal gastric branches of the anterior and posterior descending nerves of Latarjet, with preservation of the distal branches to the antrum and pylorus. Vagal division should terminate 7 cm proximal to the pylorus, whose location is marked by a prominent vein. (Figure 11-1)

Step 2: Preoperative Considerations

- HSV denervates the proximal three fourths of the stomach and the parietal cell mass. Unlike truncal and selective vagotomy, HSV does not require a concomitant gastric drainage procedure.
- By default, the celiac division of the posterior vagus and the hepatic division of the anterior vagus are preserved during HSV so that innervation to the biliary tract, and small and large bowel remains intact.
- HSV should be the procedure of choice in patients undergoing elective surgery for refractory duodenal ulcer disease, provided they do not have gastric outlet obstruction.

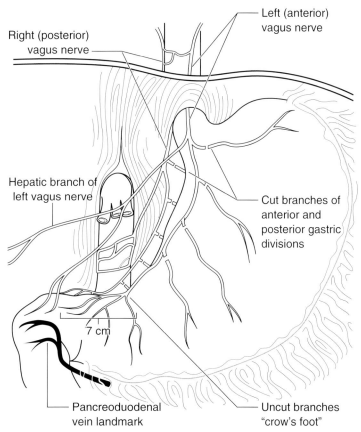

Figure 11-1

Step 3: Operative Steps

1. Positioning and Incision

+ The patient is positioned supine with both arms extended. A footboard is attached to the bed to support the patient.
+ A midline incision allows for sufficient visualization of the upper stomach and esophagus.
+ An abdominal wall retractor is placed for cephalad retraction. A sweetheart retractor attachment is placed in the midline to gently retract the junction of the esophagus and diaphragm. The patient is placed in steep reverse Trendelenburg position.
+ An orogastric tube is advanced into the proximal stomach and helps serve as a guide for palpation of the esophagus.
+ The operating surgeon stands to the patient's right.

2. Dissection

+ The gastrophrenic ligament is divided and the dissection carried over the anterior portion of the phrenoesophageal ligament towards the gastrohepatic ligament. (Figure 11-2)
+ The anterior vagus nerve is identified and encircled with a vessel loop. Superior dissection into the mediastinum ensures the division of any small vagal branches entering the stomach.
+ The gastrohepatic ligament is incised between the hepatic division and the anterior nerve of Latarjet where the surgeon inserts his or her left hand, pulling traction to the patient's right. With the assistant holding traction on the greater curvature of the stomach, the proximal gastric branches to the lesser curve are sequentially identified and transected. The dissection is ended at a point measured 7 cm proximal to the pylorus. This measurement is taken without stretching the stomach. (Figure 11-3)
+ The surgeon's right index finger is subsequently passed to the left of the esophagus in a posterior-superior direction into the mediastinum, encircling the esophagus.
+ The index finger is advanced and brought out adjacent to the right crus. The posterior vagus nerve can be palpated as a taut band on the posterior aspect of the esophagus and presented to the assistant to isolate and encircle with a second vessel loop.
+ Superior dissection away from the esophagus into the mediastinum assures division of any branching nerves.
+ After identifying and preserving the celiac branch, all gastric branches from the posterior nerve of Latarjet are proximally ligated as they course into the lesser curvature. The dissection is ended at a point that corresponds with the anterior dissection. (Figure 11-4)
+ The now denuded lesser curvature is closed with a running absorbable suture to reapproximate serosa to serosa. (Figure 11-5)

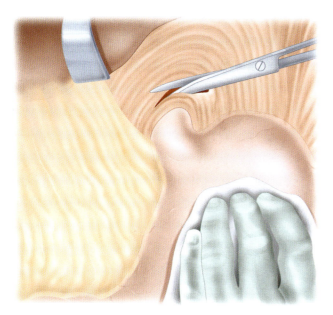

Figure 11-2

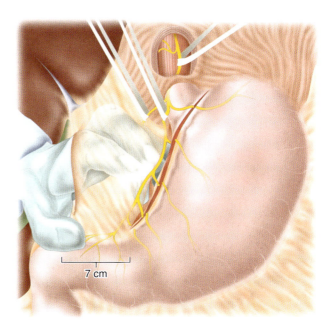

Figure 11-3

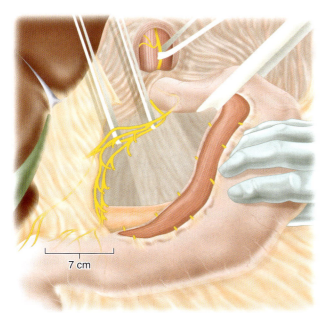

Figure 11-4

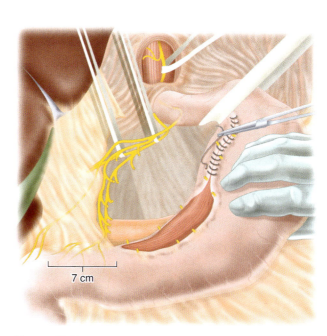

Figure 11-5

Step 4: Postoperative Care

- ◆ The patient may be started on a diet after surgery and advanced as tolerated.

Step 5: Pearls and Pitfalls

- ◆ Patients with pyloric and prepyloric ulcers have a higher ulcer recurrence rate after HSV than those with duodenal ulcers alone; thus consideration should be given to performing a truncal vagotomy with antrectomy in the former individuals.
- ◆ Reapproximating the denuded lesser curve may help to prevent ischemic necrosis of the lesser curvature and prevent the reformation of vagal innervation as well.

References

1. Donahue PE. Parietal cell vagotomy versus vagotomy-antrectomy: ulcer surgery in the modern era. *World J Surg* 2000; 24(3): 264-269.
2. Johnston D, Blackett RL. A new look at selective vagotomies. *Am J Surg* 1988; 156(5):416-427.
3. Jordan PH, Jr., Thornby J. Twenty years after parietal cell vagotomy or selective vagotomy antrectomy for treatment of duodenal ulcer. Final report. *Ann Surg* 1994; 220(3):283-293; discussion 293-296.
4. Kelly KA, Tu BN. Proximal gastric vagotomy. In: Nyhus LM, Baker RJ, Fischer JE, eds. *Mastery of surgery*. Vol. 1. Boston: Little, Brown and Company; 1997.
5. Skandalakis JE, Skandalakis PN, Skandalakis LJ. Stomach. *Surgical anatomy and technique*. New York: Springer-Verlag; 1995.
6. Skandalakis LJ, Donahue PE, Skandalakis JE. The vagus nerve and its vagaries. *Surg Clin North Am* 1993; 73(4):769-784.

CHAPTER 12

Heineke-Mikulicz Pyloroplasty

William S. Cobb IV, MD

Step 1: Surgical Anatomy

- Pyloroplasty consists of dividing the pyloric muscle and reconstructing the pyloric channel to improve gastric emptying. Following truncal vagotomy, impairment of gastric tone results in gastric stasis and requires that a drainage procedure be performed.
- To perform a pyloroplasty, ideally the anterior surface of the pylorus should have minimal fibrosis and scarring. Mobilization of the duodenum is key in order to make the operation technically feasible. If an anterior duodenal ulcer is present, the pyloroplasty incision can be modified to encompass the ulcer, still making the operation possible.
- A Heineke-Mikulicz pyloroplasty consists of a longitudinal incision through the pylorus from the distal antrum to the proximal duodenum. This incision is closed transversely to increase the diameter of the pyloric channel.

Step 2: Preoperative Considerations

- Pyloroplasty has the advantages of ease of performance, avoidance of the difficult duodenal stump, and less dissection compared to an antrectomy. It ensures drainage of the gastric antrum following vagotomy and does not alter the continuity of the gastrointestinal tract.
- For many years, pyloroplasty combined with vagotomy was considered a second option behind vagotomy and antrectomy for peptic ulcer disease due to the higher rate of failure (10% to 15%). However, with the advent of proton-pump inhibitor therapy to treat recurrences, it has become the preferred procedure in the emergent situation.
- In operations for bleeding duodenal or prepyloric ulcers, pyloroplasty is ideal if the duodenum has been opened to control bleeding.
- In the acute setting, a nasogastric tube should be placed to confirm upper gastrointestinal bleeding and to prevent aspiration. Upper endoscopy is helpful for diagnosis and potentially allows for endoscopic control of bleeding, obviating the need for an operation.
- In patients with chronic peptic ulcer disease, nutritional status should be optimized by enteral or parenteral means. It can take several days to correct nutrition and electrolytes in the patient with long-standing gastric-outlet obstruction.

◆ Preoperative preparation consists of deep vein thrombosis prophylaxis and antibiotics. Many of these patients have been on long-term proton-pump inhibitor therapy, thereby altering the acidity and bacterial flora of the gastric lumen. Preoperative antibiotics should consist of first- or second-generation cephalosporins.

Step 3: Operative Steps

1. Incision

◆ An upper midline incision provides adequate exposure for most gastric procedures. In the emergent setting, this approach provides the quickest and driest entry into the abdominal cavity. Alternatively, a left subcostal incision may be used; however, this is more painful and can result in a higher rate of hernia formation.

◆ The upper midline incision may be extended superiorly to the xiphoid process for exposure of the esophageal hiatus. The cartilaginous xiphoid should not be cauterized to avoid heterotopic ossification.

◆ Once the peritoneum is entered, the falciform ligament should be divided to allow for upward retraction of the left lateral lobe of the liver.

2. Dissection

◆ Typically, a Kocher maneuver is required to perform a pyloroplasty. The peritoneum just lateral to the second portion of the duodenum is incised. (Figure 12-1AB) If mobilization of the duodenum is feasible and the anterior surface of the pylorus is minimally involved, a pyloroplasty is reasonable.

◆ The pylorus is identified with the pyloric vein of Mayo as a landmark. (Figure 12-2)

◆ Two traction sutures are placed on the anterior surface of the pylorus approximately 1 cm apart. Traction sutures should incorporate the pyloric vein so as to partially control the subsequent bleeding. The longitudinal incision is made between the traction sutures. The length of the incision should be approximately 5 cm with a 2.5- to 3-cm extension onto both the duodenum and antrum. (Figure 12-3) Bleeding is controlled with cautery or suture ligatures.

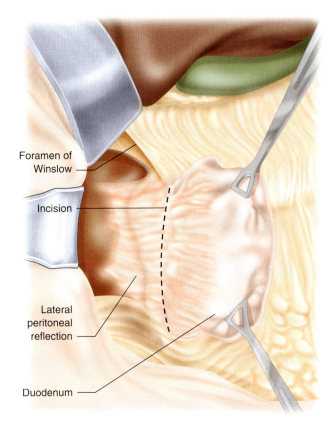

Foramen of
Winslow

Incision

Lateral
peritoneal
reflection

Duodenum

A

Figure 12-1

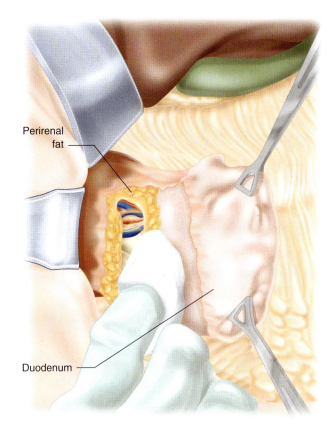

Perirenal
fat

Duodenum

B

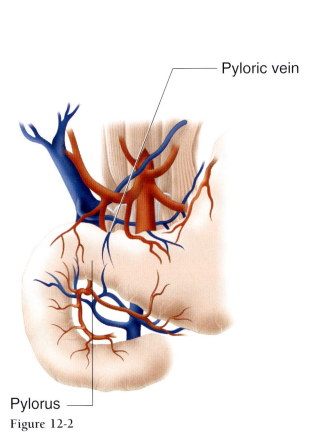

Pyloric vein

Pylorus

Figure 12-2

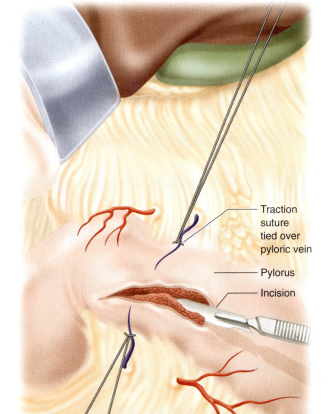

Traction
suture
tied over
pyloric vein

Pylorus

Incision

Figure 12-3

- The original description of the Heineke-Mikulicz pyloroplasty outlined a two-layer closure (Figure 12-4AB); however, this technique may cause infolding of additional tissue, decreasing the diameter of the opening.
- The Weinberg modification describes a single layer of interrupted suture that provides good closure. 3-0 polyglactin 910 or silk suture on a tapered needle works well. Full-thickness sutures are important for good approximation of the serosa and inversion of the mucosa. A Gambee stitch accomplishes a nice single-layer closure approximating the mucosa. (Figure 12-5AB)
- The first suture is placed at the midpoint of the suture line. Proceed with closure from one corner to the midpoint and then from the other corner to the midpoint. Wait to tie the sutures until all are placed. The edges of the tissue can be better manipulated to allow for better visualization so that good seromuscular bites are achieved.

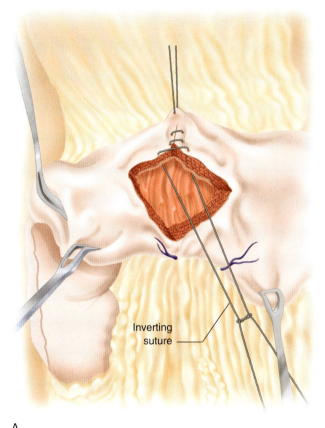

Inverting suture

A

Figure 12-4

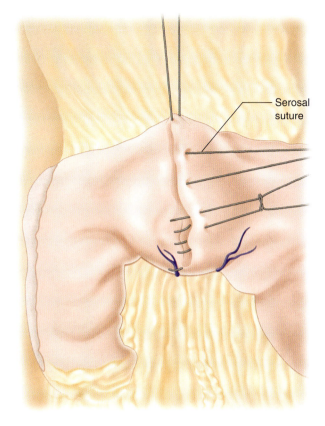

Serosal suture

B

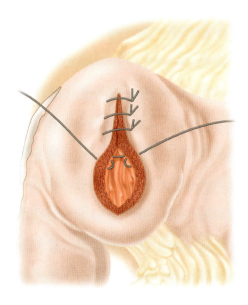

A

Figure 12-5

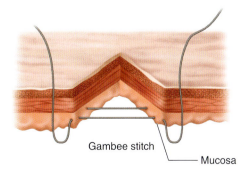

Gambee stitch

Mucosa

B

- Alternatively, a stapling device can be used to create the pyloroplasty. Allis clamps are used to grasp the cut ends of the tissue, everting them mucosa to mucosa. A noncutting linear stapler is placed just deep to the line of the Allis clamps. The stapler is fired and tissue excised with a scalpel. (Figure 12-6AB) Bleeding from the staple line is best controlled with suture ligatures.
- When an ulcer is present on the anterior duodenal wall, the Heineke-Mikulicz pyloroplasty can be modified to incorporate the ulcer in the incision. The Horsley modification excises the anterior ulcer. (Figure 12-7AB) This technique is advantageous if the ulcer is limited to the anterior surface or if the ulcer has thinned out the duodenal wall. If the ulcer is more extensive and the tissue is not suitable for suturing, a Jaboulay gastroduodenostomy should be performed.

3. Closing

- The position of the nasogastric tube is confirmed intraoperatively. The tip of the tube should be in the distal body of the stomach and not in the area of the suture line. Alternatively, a gastrostomy can be performed.
- Once bleeding has been controlled, the incision is closed with running absorbable, monofilamented suture.
- Drains are not typically left in the operative field.

Step 4: Postoperative Care

- A nasogastric tube is left postoperatively for gastric decompression. The tube can be removed when output is less than a liter per day, and the patient is not nauseated.
- Once the nasogastric tube has been removed, feeding is begun slowly with liquids progressing to a regular diet. High carbohydrate loads are best avoided to limit dumping symptoms.
- Occasionally, delayed gastric emptying requires prolonged tube decompression. A contrast study via the nasogastric tube should demonstrate anatomical patency. In cases of persistent nausea and vomiting with inability to remove the nasogastric tube, an endoscopic gastrostomy tube placement is preferable to reoperation. Through a gastrostomy, a feeding jejunostomy can be fed for enteral nutrition. In cases where there is a small gastric remnant, total parenteral nutrition is an option.
- Suture line leaks may create a potentially fatal situation. There should be a high level of awareness for such problems within the first 5 to 6 postoperative days. Leaks are usually associated with tachycardia, increasing abdominal pain, fever, distention, and leukocytosis. Prompt investigation with abdominal films, contrasted CT, or contrast upper GI series should be undertaken. While controlled leaks may be managed nonoperatively, most require reoperation. Irrigation and drainage, decompression of the leaking segment, closure or intubation of the leak, and feeding jejunostomy are important facets of management.

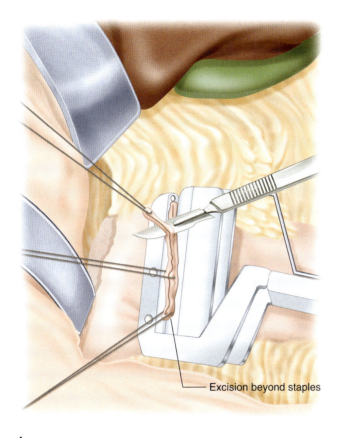

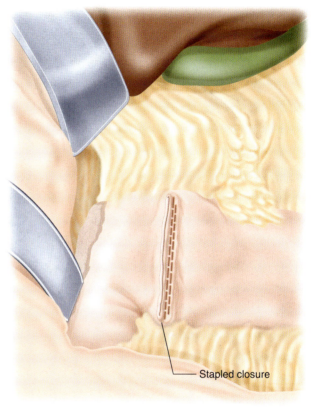

A

Figure 12-6

B

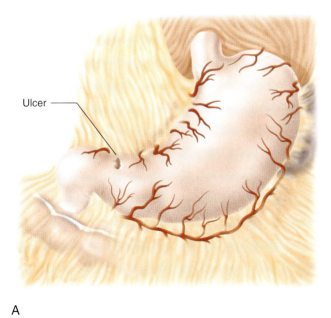

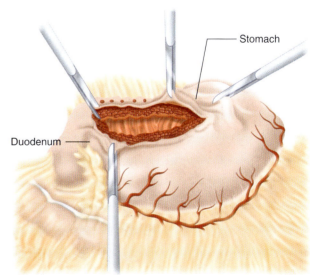

A

Figure 12-7

B

Step 5: Pearls and Pitfalls

- If there is difficulty in identifying the pylorus, a small incision can be made on the gastric side of the presumed pyloric location. The finger can be inserted into the gastric lumen and palpation from the inside can usually determine the exact location of the pyloric ring. (Figure 12-8)
- To ensure adequate closure of the incision, extending the incision more onto the gastric side may provide better alignment when the incision is closed transversely. The total length of the incision should be at least 5 cm but not more than 7 cm.
- The gastric wall is much thicker than the duodenum making it difficult to prevent eversion of the mucosa between the sutures. Interrupted seromuscular stitches or Lembert sutures can help minimize the discrepancy.
- Tags of the omentum can be used to buttress the suture line following a pyloroplasty. The tails of the sutures on each end of the completed pyloroplasty can be used to loosely secure an omental flap to prevent leakage of the suture line.

References

1. Grabowski MW, Dempsey DT. Pyloroplasty (Heineke-Mikulicz and Finney) operation for bleeding duodenal ulcer. In: Scott-Conner CE, ed. *Chassin's operative strategy in general surgery.* 3rd ed. New York: Springer; 2002.
2. Martin CJ, Kennedy T. Reconstruction of the pylorus. *World J Surg* 1982; 6:221-225.
3. Soreide K, Sarr MG, Soreide JA. Pyloroplasty for benign gastric outlet obstruction-indication and techniques. *Scand J Surg* 2006; 95(1):11-16.
4. Soybel DI, Zinner MJ. Stomach and duodenum: operative procedures. In: Zinner MJ, Schwartz SI, Ellis H, eds. *Maingot's abdominal operations.* 10th ed. Stamford, CT: Appleton & Lange; 1997.

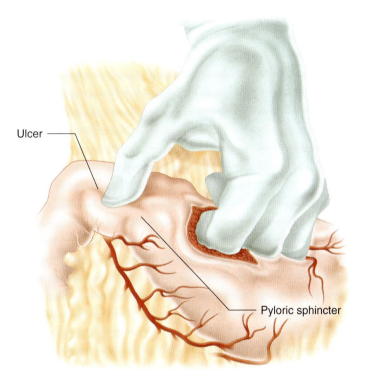

Ulcer

Pyloric sphincter

Figure 12-8

CHAPTER 13

FINNEY PYLOROPLASTY

William S. Cobb IV, MD

Step 1: Surgical Anatomy

- The Finney pyloroplasty is preferred when a longer incision on the duodenum is required to control bleeding. A fibrotic duodenum may require closure with a Finney pyloroplasty as well.
- When scarring of the pylorus and duodenal bulb prohibits a tension-free patulous Heineke-Mikulicz pyloroplasty, a Finney-type closure can be used. The Finney pyloroplasty is essentially a side-to-side gastroduodenostomy.

Step 2: Preoperative Considerations

- In the acute setting, a nasogastric tube should be placed to confirm upper gastrointestinal bleeding and to prevent aspiration. Upper endoscopy is helpful for diagnosis and potentially allows for endoscopic control of bleeding, obviating the need for an operation.
- In chronic patients with peptic ulcer disease, nutritional status should be optimized by enteral or parenteral means. It can take several days to correct nutrition and electrolytes in the patient with long-term gastric-outlet obstruction.
- Patients requiring an operation for long-term outlet obstruction often have dilatation and elongation of the stomach. A Finney pyloroplasty is preferred in this instance because it provides better drainage of the stomach.
- Preoperative preparation consists of deep vein thrombosis prophylaxis and antibiotics. Many of these patients have been on long-term proton-pump inhibitor therapy, thereby altering the acidity and bacterial flora of the gastric lumen. Preoperative antibiotics should consist of first- or second-generation cephalosporins.

Step 3: Operative Steps

1. Incision

- An upper midline incision provides adequate exposure for most gastric procedures. In the emergent setting, this approach provides the quickest and driest entry into the abdominal cavity. Alternatively, a left subcostal incision may be used; however, this is more painful and results in a higher rate of hernia formation.
- The upper midline incision may be extended superiorly to the xiphoid process for exposure of the esophageal hiatus. The cartilaginous xiphoid should not be cauterized to avoid heterotopic ossification.
- Once the peritoneum is entered, the falciform ligament should be divided to allow for upward retraction of the left lateral lobe of the liver.

2. Dissection

- Unlike the Heineke-Mikulicz pyloroplasty, the incision for the Finney pyloroplasty is closer to the greater curvature on the stomach side and onto the medial aspect of the duodenum on the pancreatic side. This incision location relieves tension on the anterior suture line. (Figure 13-1)
- A row of interrupted 3-0 silk or polyglactin 910 sutures are placed to approximate the greater curvature to the superior portion of the proximal duodenum. It is preferable if the sutures are placed prior to making the pyloroplasty incision. (Figure 13-2)
- An inverted U-shaped incision is made approximately 5 mm from the suture line. This incision is continued full thickness. The mucosa of the duodenum and gastric antrum should be easily visible. (Figure 13-3)

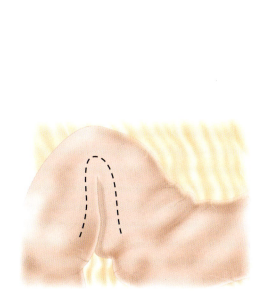

Figure 13-1

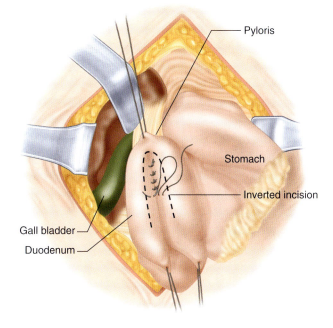

Figure 13-2

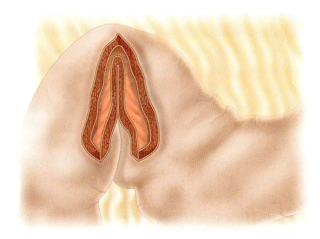

Figure 13-3

- The mucosa is reapproximated by starting at the inferior layer with a 3-0 polyglactin suture. The suture is run caudally in a locking fashion. When the end of the incision is reached, the suture is passed from the inside-out on the gastric side. (Figure 13-4)
- The anterior mucosal layer is closed with same suture with a continuous Connell suture. (Figure 13-5) An additional seromuscular, Lembert layer of 4-0 silk or polyglactin is placed on the anterior serosal closure. (Figure 13-6)
- At the completion of the Finney pyloroplasty, the lumen should accommodate two fingers.

3. Closing

- The position of the nasogastric tube is confirmed intraoperatively. The tip of the tube should be in the distal body of the stomach and not in the area of the suture line. Alternatively, a gastrostomy can be performed.
- Once bleeding has been controlled, the incision is closed with running absorbable, monofilamented suture.
- Drains are not typically left in the operative field.

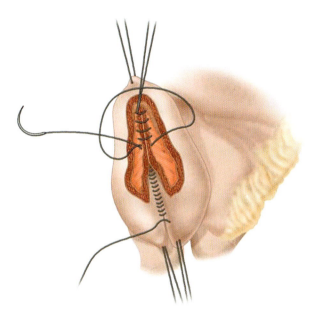

Figure 13-4

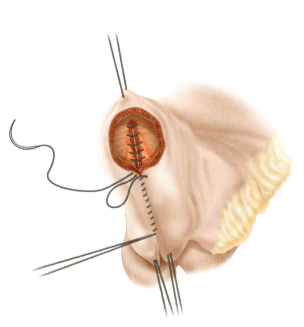

Figure 13-5

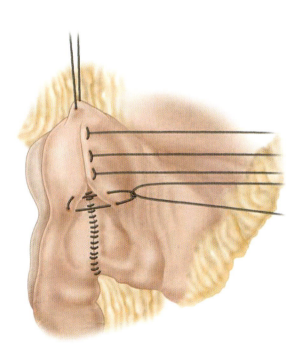

Figure 13-6

Step 4: Postoperative Care

- A nasogastric tube is left postoperatively for gastric decompression. The tube can be removed when output is less than a liter per day, and the patient is not nauseated.
- Once the nasogastric tube has been removed, feeding is begun slowly with liquids progressing to a regular diet. High carbohydrate loads are best avoided to limit dumping symptoms.
- Occasionally, delayed gastric emptying requires prolonged tube decompression. A contrast study via the nasogastric tube should demonstrate anatomical patency. In cases of persistent nausea and vomiting with inability to remove the nasogastric tube, an endoscopic gastrostomy tube placement is preferable to reoperation. Through a gastrostomy, a feeding jejunostomy can be fed for enteral nutrition. In cases where there is a small gastric remnant, total parenteral nutrition is an option.
- Suture line leaks may create a potentially fatal situation. There should be a high level of awareness for such problems within the first 5 to 6 postoperative days. Leaks are usually associated with tachycardia, increasing abdominal pain, fever, distention, and leukocytosis. Prompt investigation with abdominal films, contrasted CT, or contrast upper GI series should be undertaken. While controlled leaks may be managed nonoperatively, most require reoperation. Irrigation and drainage, decompression of the leaking segment, closure or intubation of the leak, and feeding jejunostomy are important facets of management.

Step 5: Pearls and Pitfalls

◆ A Finney pyloroplasty should be considered when the ulcer is located distal on the duodenum. When the ulcer is present at a distance beyond 4 to 5 cm, a Finney-type pyloroplasty is preferable to a Heineke-Mikulicz.
◆ To reduce tension on the suture line with a Finney pyloroplasty, a generous Kocher maneuver is required to allow for extensive duodenal mobilization. A single-layer closure of the gastroenterotomy is preferred to two layers to reduce tension.

References

1. Grabowski MW, Dempsey DT. Pyloroplasty (Heineke-Mikulicz and Finney) operation for bleeding duodenal ulcer. In: Scott-Conner CE, ed. *Chassin's operative strategy in general surgery*. 3rd ed. New York: Springer; 2002.
2. Martin CJ, Kennedy T. Reconstruction of the pylorus. *World J Surg* 1982; 6:221.
3. Soybel DI, Zinner MJ. Stomach and duodenum: operative procedures. In: Zinner MJ, Schwartz SI, Ellis H, eds. *Maingot's abdominal operations*. 10th ed. Stamford, CT: Appleton & Lange; 1997.

CHAPTER 14

JABOULAY PYLOROPLASTY

William S. Cobb IV, MD

Step 1: Clinical Anatomy

- Jaboulay "pyloroplasty" is actually a gastroduodenostomy between the antrum of the stomach and the duodenum. The pylorus is not technically incised. (Figure 14-1)
- This operation results in a large opening between the distal stomach and duodenum and avoids the inflammatory process in the pyloric area.

Step 2: Preoperative Considerations

- Jaboulay gastroduodenostomy combined with a truncal vagotomy is best suited in the treatment of gastric-outlet obstruction from a duodenal ulcer. The Jaboulay gastroduodenostomy effectively improves gastric emptying.
- The Jaboulay gastroduodenostomy has the advantages of relatively easy exposure and dissection. The technique avoids the dissection of inflamed or friable peripyloric tissue. There is no need to oversew or disturb the ulcer base if no active bleeding has occurred.

Step 3: Operative Steps

1. Incision

- An upper midline incision provides adequate exposure for most gastric procedures. In the emergent setting, this approach provides the quickest and driest entry into the abdominal cavity. Alternatively, a left subcostal incision may be used; however, this is more painful and results in a higher rate of hernia formation.
- The upper midline incision may be extended superiorly to the xiphoid process for exposure of the esophageal hiatus. The cartilaginous xiphoid should not be cauterized to avoid heterotopic ossification.

Jaboulay

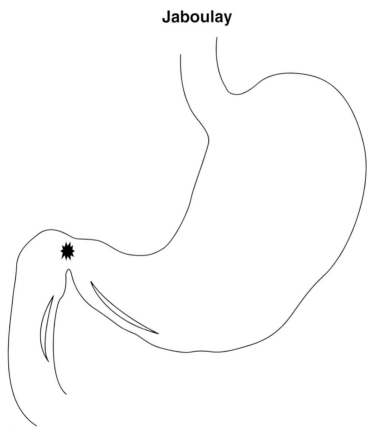

Figure 14-1

♦ Once the peritoneum is entered, the falciform ligament should be divided to allow for upward retraction of the left lateral lobe of the liver.

2. Dissection

♦ A Kocher maneuver is performed by mobilizing the lateral aspect of the second portion of the duodenum. The first two fingers of the left hand can be used to bluntly open up the plane behind the duodenum. A scissor motion can help to open up the retroperitoneal and retropancreatic space.
♦ The antrum of the stomach and the duodenum are aligned by placing a traction suture just proximal to the pylorus along the greater curve of the stomach. This site is approximated to an area of the duodenum just distal to scarred pylorus. A second traction suture is placed more proximal on the stomach along the greater curve and more distal on the duodenum approximately 7 to 9 cm from the first suture. (Figure 14-2)
♦ The posterior interrupted layer is placed first. Silk or polyglactin 910 (3-0) is used to approximate the serosal surfaces of the stomach and duodenum. (Figure 14-3)
♦ The stomach and duodenum are then opened. Once hemostasis is achieved, an inner, continuous, absorbable layer (polyglactin or polydioxanone) is placed and carried anteriorly. A double-armed suture is placed at the midpoint of the posterior opening and continued cephalad and caudad. (Figure 14-4) The anastomosis is completed with an interrupted layer of silk or polyglactin suture utilizing a Lembert stitch. (Figure 14-5)

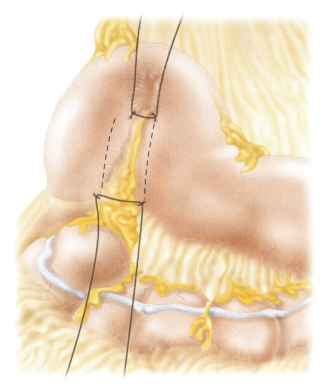

Figure 14-2

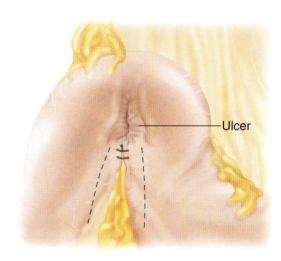

Figure 14-3

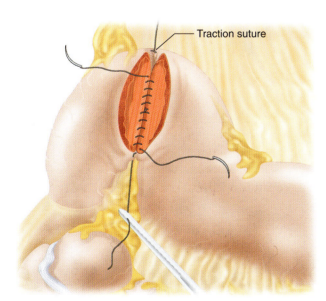

Figure 14-4

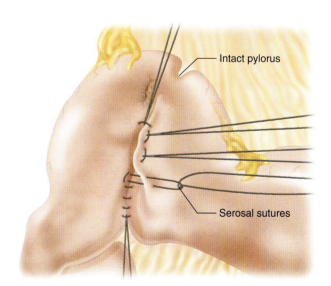

Figure 14-5

3. Closing

- The position of the nasogastric tube is confirmed intraoperatively. The tip of the tube should be in the distal body of the stomach and not in the area of the suture line. Alternatively, a gastrostomy can be performed.
- Once bleeding has been controlled, the incision is closed with running absorbable, monofilamented suture.
- Drains are not typically left in the operative field.

Step 4: Postoperative Care

- A nasogastric tube is left postoperatively for gastric decompression. The tube can be removed when output is less than a liter per day, and the patient is not nauseated.
- Once the nasogastric tube has been removed, feeding is begun slowly with liquids progressing to a regular diet. High carbohydrate loads are best avoided to limit dumping symptoms.
- Occasionally, delayed gastric emptying requires prolonged tube decompression. A contrast study via the nasogastric tube should demonstrate anatomical patency. In cases of persistent nausea and vomiting with inability to remove the nasogastric tube, an endoscopic gastrostomy tube placement is preferable to reoperation. Through a gastrostomy, a feeding jejunostomy can be fed for enteral nutrition. In cases where there is a small gastric remnant, total parenteral nutrition is an option.
- Suture line leaks may create a potentially fatal situation. There should be a high level of awareness for such problems within the first 5 to 6 postoperative days. Leaks are usually associated with tachycardia, increasing abdominal pain, fever, distention, and leukocytosis. Prompt investigation with abdominal films, contrasted CT, or contrast upper GI series should be undertaken. While controlled leaks may be managed nonoperatively, most require reoperation. Irrigation and drainage, decompression of the leaking segment, closure or intubation of the leak, and feeding jejunostomy are important facets of management.

Step 5: Pearls And Pitfalls

- Following the Kocher maneuver it is beneficial to identify the middle colic vessels, which can swing down over the duodenum in order to avoid injury during dissection.
- The fine tip of an electrocautery pencil works well to create the gastrotomy and duodenotomy. It provides better hemostasis than the scalpel, and the fine tip minimizes cautery damage.

References

1. Farris JM, Smith GK. Long-term appraisal of the treatment of gastric ulcer in situ by vagotomy and pyloroplasty with a note on the Jaboulay procedure. *Am J Surg*, 1973; 126(2):292-299.
2. Sawyers, JL. Selective vagotomy and pyloroplasty. In: Nyhus LM, Baker RJ, Fischer JE, eds. *Mastery of surgery*. 3rd ed. Boston: Little, Brown and Co.; 1997.

CHAPTER 15

ANTRECTOMY

William S. Cobb IV, MD

Step 1: Surgical Anatomy

- Surgery of the stomach and duodenum requires an understanding of both the blood supply of the stomach and duodenum and the anatomical relationships to the pancreas and spleen. (Figure 15-1)

Step 2: Preoperative Considerations

- The most common indications for antrectomy or distal gastrectomy are duodenal ulcer disease, gastric ulcer, and benign gastric tumors. Relative contraindications include cirrhosis, extensive scarring of the proximal duodenum, and previous surgery on the proximal duodenum.
- When performed in combination with a truncal vagotomy, antrectomy is the gold standard in reducing acid secretion and recurrence when compared to vagotomy, pyloroplasty, and highly selective vagotomy. However, the low recurrence rates must be weighed against the postgastrectomy and postvagotomy complications that occur in approximately 20% of patients. In the H. pylori era, antrectomy is performed infrequently in patients with peptic ulcer disease.
- Antrectomy with Billroth I reconstruction (gastroduodenostomy) is the most physiologic gastric resection as it restores the normal continuity. Combined with vagotomy, antrectomy allows for retention of 50% of the stomach with the lowest recurrence rate of all ulcer procedures. (Figure 15-2)
- In the malnourished patient, especially female, antrectomy leaves enough of a gastric reservoir to allow for maintenance of adequate postoperative nutrition. Constructing the gastroduodenal anastomosis to approximate the size of the pylorus usually delays gastric emptying and reduces problems with postgastrectomy dumping.
- The patient's nutritional status must be adequately assessed. Preoperative labs should include prealbumin and albumin levels.
- In the acute setting, electrolytes must be corrected. When chronic nausea and vomiting is present, alkalosis must be corrected and potassium levels restored.

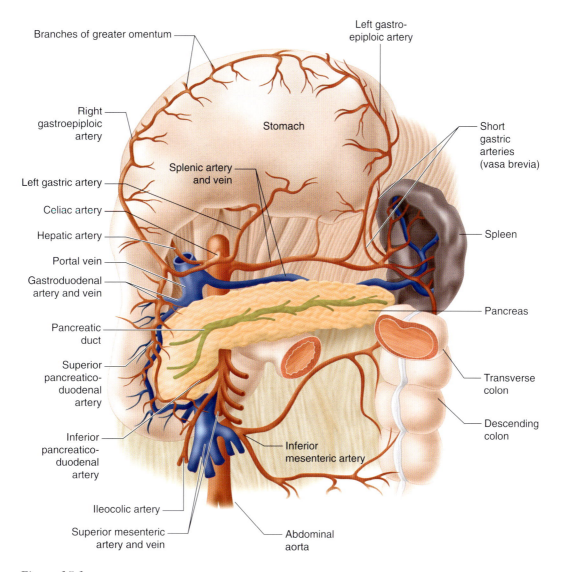

Branches of greater omentum

Left gastro-epiploic artery

Right gastroepiploic artery

Stomach

Short gastric arteries (vasa brevia)

Splenic artery and vein

Left gastric artery

Celiac artery

Hepatic artery

Spleen

Portal vein

Gastroduodenal artery and vein

Pancreatic duct

Pancreas

Superior pancreatico-duodenal artery

Transverse colon

Inferior pancreatico-duodenal artery

Descending colon

Inferior mesenteric artery

Ileocolic artery

Superior mesenteric artery and vein

Abdominal aorta

Figure 15-1

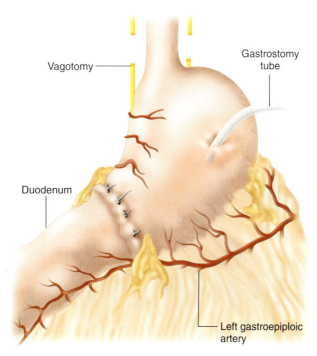

Vagotomy

Gastrostomy tube

Duodenum

Left gastroepiploic artery

Figure 15-2

Step 3: Operative Steps

1. **Incision**

 ◆ An upper midline incision works well to provide adequate exposure to the stomach. This incision can be extended to the xiphoid to gain access to the esophageal hiatus for vagotomy. In patients with a barrel-shaped chest, a subcostal incision may provide slightly better access to the foregut. However, dividing the muscle results in more potential wound problems and more dissection time.
 ◆ Once the peritoneum is entered, the falciform ligament should be divided to allow for upward retraction of the left lateral lobe of the liver.

2. **Dissection**

 ◆ The first step of antrectomy for ulcer disease is to evaluate the duodenum for possible resection and the possibility of a difficult duodenal stump closure. This determination is difficult by inspection alone. A marked fibrotic or edematous anterior duodenal wall suggests that duodenal closure will be difficult. Extensive edema or fibrosis of the pylorus, pancreas, and hepatoduodenal ligaments is a relative contraindication to antrectomy.
 ◆ Extensive duodenal mobilization is a necessity for a Billroth I reconstruction. The peritoneum along the lateral border of the second portion of the duodenum is incised and a Kocher maneuver performed. Typically, the duodenum can be retracted medially with the left hand, and the peritoneal attachments are swept away with the blunt finger or gauze. Again, the middle colic vessels course over the second portion of the duodenum and may be encountered suddenly. The hepatic flexure should be directed caudally and medially to identify the middle colic vessels early. (Figure 15-3)
 ◆ The avascular hepatogastric ligament is incised to the right of the lesser curve. This maneuver allows for passage of the left forefinger behind the antrum, emerging posterior to the gastroepiploic arcade along the greater curvature. The omentum is elevated off of the transverse mesocolon and opened, thus avoiding injury to the middle colic vessels. (Figure 15-4) The branches of the gastroepiploic arcade going to the greater curve are sequentially divided with clamps and ties. This dissection is continued along the greater curve until a point that is approximately halfway from the pylorus and the diaphragm. (Figure 15-5) The distal segment of the gastroepiploic arcade is dissected off of the antrum. Care should be taken as the fragile veins near the origin of the right gastroepiploic vessels can be easily torn. During this dissection, the congenital attachments of the pancreas to the back wall of the antrum can be taken down to completely mobilize the distal half of the greater curve.
 ◆ A site along the lesser curve is identified just proximal to the third prominent vein. This point is roughly halfway between the esophagogastric junction and the pylorus and is a good estimation of the upper extent of antral mucosa. A hemostat is inserted between the lesser curve and the adjacent vascular bundle in this area. The left gastric vessels are divided between two clamps. (Figure 15-6) Ligatures of 0 silk or polyglactin 910 are used to control the cut ends of the vessels. Preferably, at least a 1-cm stump of gastric artery is left beyond each tie. There may be additional small gastric veins that require additional ties.

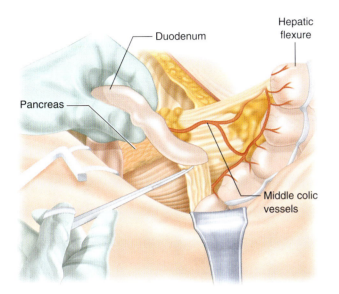

Figure 15-3

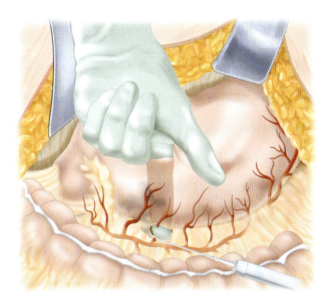

Figure 15-4

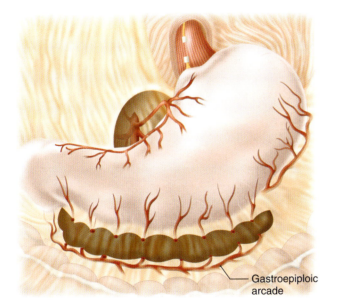

Figure 15-5

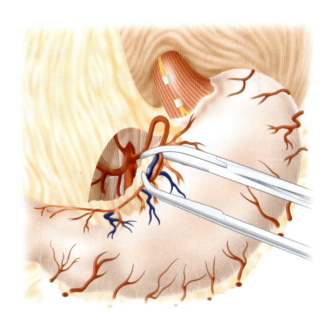

Figure 15-6

- The omentum is retracted upward, and the posterior wall of the stomach is freed up from the capsule of the pancreas. Any adhesions encountered should be taken down sharply. If a posterior ulcer is present, there may be erosion into the capsule of the pancreas. The attachments can be broken up with the thumb and forefinger, leaving the ulcer crater on the capsule of the pancreas. (Figure 15-7) All gastric ulcers should be biopsied to rule out the presence of malignancy.
- At this point, extensive mobilization of the duodenum and stomach is ensured. No commitment to resection has been made. Once it appears feasible to perform an antrectomy, the surgeon proceeds with division of the stomach and duodenum.
- Combined with a complete vagotomy, no more than half of the stomach needs to be removed. The stomach may be divided with the single firing of a linear stapler typically 90 mm in length, with either 3.5- or 4.8-mm staple heights. This technique sets things up better for a stapled gastrointestinal anastomosis. (Figure 15-8) For a hand-sewn reconstruction, longitudinal serrated visceral clamps are placed at 90-degree angles to the greater curve for a distance of about 3 to 4 cm. The amount of tissue in the clamp should correspond to the desired size of anastomotic opening for the gastroduodenostomy or gastrojejunostomy. The gastric wall is divided between the clamps. A linear stapler is used to divide the remaining portion of the stomach on the lesser curve side. (Figure 15-9) An additional Allen clamp is placed distal to the stapler, and the stomach divided flush with the stapler. The cut end of the stomach may be cauterized for hemostasis. It is preferable to use absorbable staple-line reinforcement to minimize bleeding. An interrupted layer of 4-0 silk or polyglactin can be used to invert the staple line of the gastric

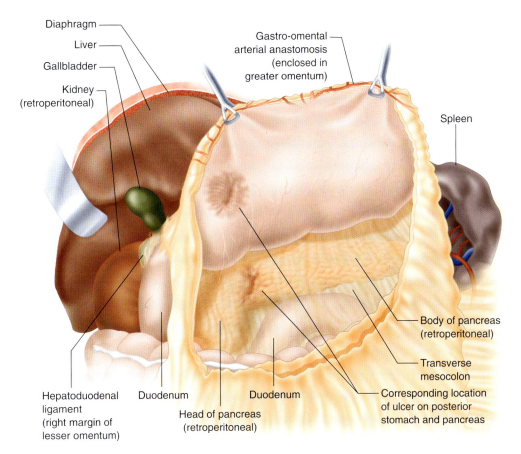

Diaphragm

Liver

Gallbladder

Kidney
(retroperitoneal)

Gastro-omental
arterial anastomosis
(enclosed in
greater omentum)

Spleen

Body of pancreas
(retroperitoneal)

Transverse
mesocolon

Corresponding location
of ulcer on posterior
stomach and pancreas

Hepatoduodenal
ligament
(right margin of
lesser omentum)

Duodenum

Head of pancreas
(retroperitoneal)

Duodenum

Figure 15-7

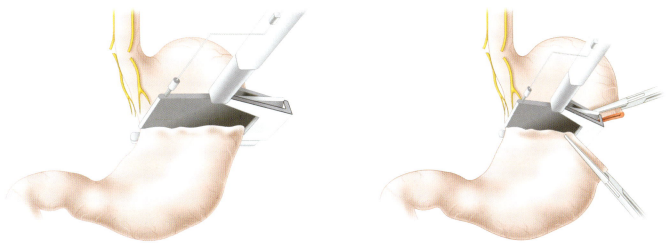

Figure 15-8

Figure 15-9

pouch using a Lembert suture. When a stapling device is not used or available, the lesser curve is divided between two Allen clamps. A 3-0 polyglactin suture is used to close the gastric pouch in layers, starting on the lesser curve side. The suture needle is passed back and forth just deep to the Allen clamp to make a running horizontal mattress stitch. When the base of the Allen clamp is reached, the same suture is run back to the lesser curve using a running, locked suture and tied to its point of origin. The mucosa is then inverted with an interrupted, Lembert layer of 4-0 silk or polyglactin. (Figure 15-10ABC)

- Attention is directed to division of the duodenum. In the absence of significant fibrosis and scarring, the duodenum is mobilized and prepared for a Billroth I anastomosis. At least 1 to 1.5 cm of duodenal wall must be cleared of fat and vessels on both the superior and inferior edge. The right gastric artery is identified and ligated. (Figure 15-11) The resected gastric specimen is retracted anteriorly to expose the posterior wall of the duodenum and anterior surface of the pancreas. There will be several (five to six) small perforating vessels from the pancreas to the duodenum. These need to be ligated with 4-0 sutures between fine-tipped hemostats. If the vessel retracts into the substance of the pancreas, a mattress suture of 4-0 silk or polyglactin can be used to control the bleeding. (Figure 15-12)

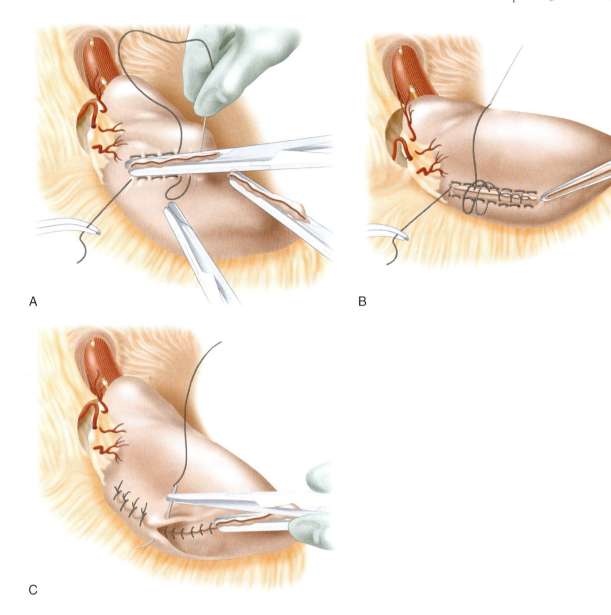

A

B

C

Figure 15-10

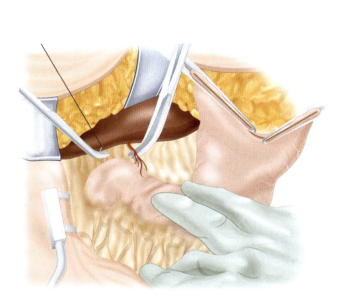

Figure 15-11

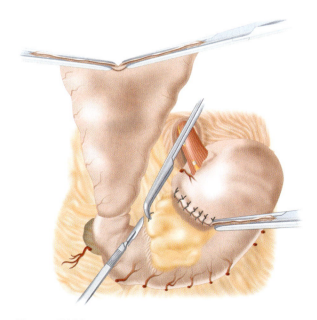

Figure 15-12

- Proper and safe division of the duodenum is paramount but sometimes quite difficult, especially in the presence of posterior penetrating duodenal ulcers. The anterior wall of the duodenum just distal to the ulcer scar is divided first. This cut is made with a scalpel as close to the pylorus as the ulcer allows. The posterior wall of the duodenum is then incised from internal to external under direct visualization. (Figure 15-13) If a posterior penetrating ulcer is present immediately distal to the pylorus, the distal duodenum can usually be freed up enough to perform an anastomosis once the duodenum is divided. If a posterior duodenal ulcer is present more distally (beyond 2.5 cm), the posterior wall of the duodenum will need to be left attached to the ulcer bed so that a modified closure of the complex duodenal stump can be performed.

- Once the duodenum is divided, the surgeon should identify the ampulla of Vater. The right index finger is inserted into the duodenal lumen to palpate the ampulla. This structure is typically 5 cm from the cut edge of the duodenum and 7 cm from the pylorus. Once the exact entry point of the common duct is noted, the surgeon can more comfortably proceed with gastrointestinal reconstruction.

- At this point, the surgeon must decide which anastomosis to perform. There are few instances in which an end-to-end gastroduodenal anastomosis cannot be performed. The anastomosis should never be forced. If reestablishing gastroduodenal continuity will be difficult, a gastrojejunal anastomosis should be performed.

- For an end-to-end gastroduodenal anastomosis, the Allen clamp previously placed on the cut end of the greater curve portion of the stomach should have a length of tissue roughly equal to the cut end of the duodenum. The corner sutures are placed first using the Cushing technique. A posterior layer of interrupted 4-0 silk or polyglactin Lembert sutures is placed. Care should be taken not to incorporate large bites of tissue, to reduce incidence of postoperative obstruction. (Figure 15-14) Remove the Allen clamp. A double-armed 4-0 polyglactin suture is placed at the midpoint of the posterior wall and tied. The mucosal layer is closed in both directions using a continuous, locking stitch for hemostasis. Anteriorly, the sutures are continued using a Connell stitch. The anterior suture line is reinforced with an interrupted 4-0 silk or polyglactin Lembert stitches. (Figure 15-15ABC) At the "angle of sorrow" where the gastric suture line meets the superior edge of the duodenum, a crown stitch is placed, incorporating the seromuscular layer of the anterior wall of the gastric pouch, the posterior wall of the gastric pouch, and the wall of the duodenum. (Figure 15-16) The completed anastomosis should accommodate the thumb of the surgeon. An omental patch is loosely secured over the anastomosis. The tails of the corner sutures can be used to secure the omentum before they are cut.

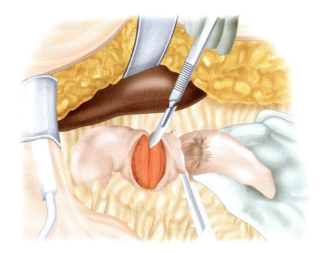

Figure 15-13

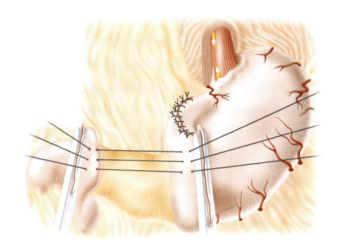

Figure 15-14

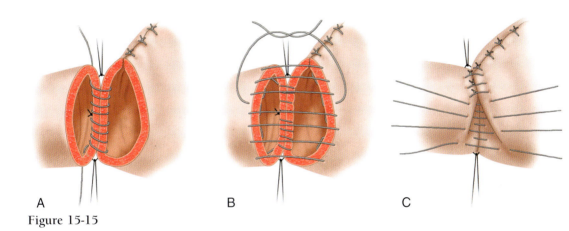

A   B   C

Figure 15-15

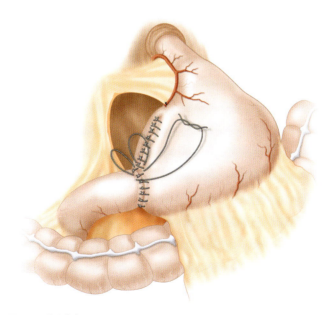

Figure 15-16

◆ A gastrojejunostomy, or Billroth II reconstruction, can be performed either in a hand sewn or stapled manner. An antecolic anastomosis is preferable, although a retrocolic reconstruction can be fashioned by bringing the jejunum through the transverse mesocolon. An area of the jejunum approximately 12 to 15 cm from the ligament of Treitz is chosen. The loop of jejunum is brought up to the greater curve side of the divided stomach that is contained in the Allen clamp. The antimesenteric border of the jejunum is marked with an ink pen or scored with the back of a scalpel blade. The posterior seromuscular layer is placed first in an interrupted fashion using 4-0 silk or polyglactin 910 suture. The mark on the jejunum ensures that this layer is placed in a straight line. (Figure 15-17) The tails of the two corner sutures are left long and used as traction sutures for the remaining anastomosis. Excess stomach contained in the Allen clamp is resected flush with the clamp, and the clamp removed. A full thickness jejunostomy is created with pen electrocautery at a site along the mark. The tips of a hemostat are inserted into the jejunal lumen and the jejunostomy is opened up for a distance that is slightly less than the gastric opening. The mucosal layers are approximated with a double-armed 3-0 polyglactin suture. The suture is placed at the midpoint of the posterior layer and tied. The suture is then run in a continuous, locked fashion toward each lateral margin. (Figure 15-18) The anterior mucosal layer is completed with a continuous Connell stitch. The two strands are tied to each other at the anterior midpoint. A second, interrupted layer of Lembert sutures are placed using 4-0 silk or polyglactin. (Figure 15-19) At the medial margin, a crown stitch (as described before in the gastroduodenostomy technique) is placed in the crotch of the gastric and jejunal anastomosis. (Figure 15-20)

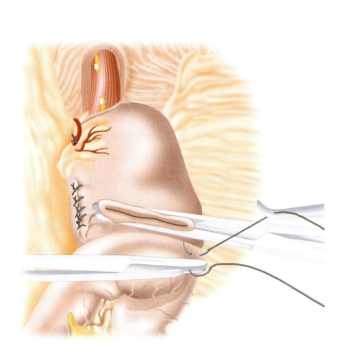

Figure 15-17

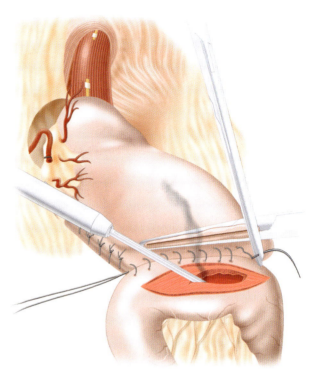

Figure 15-18

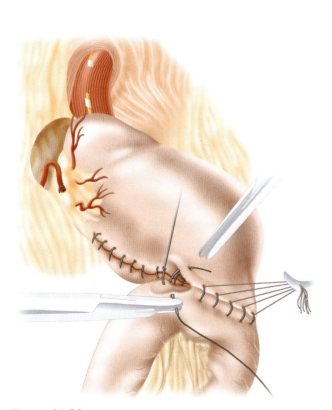

Figure 15-19

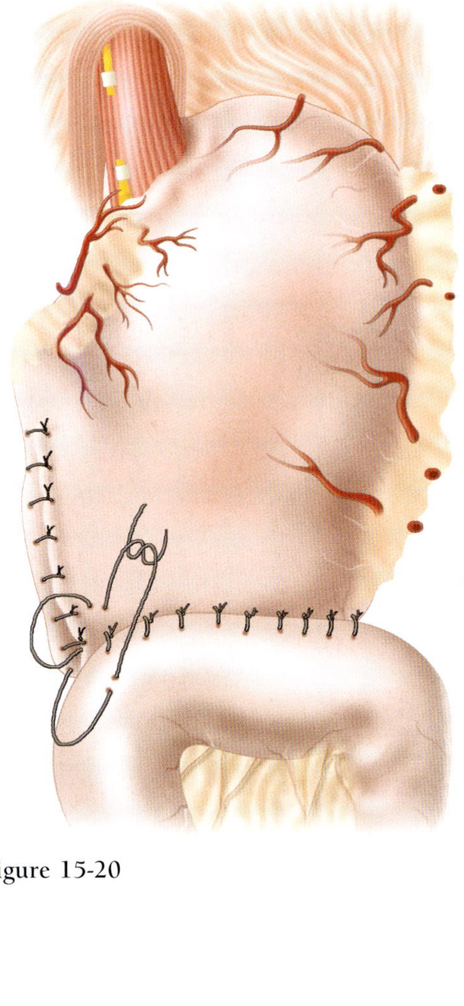

Figure 15-20

♦ In the era of laparoscopy and stapling technology, many surgeons are more comfortable with a stapled anastomosis. In this case, the entire stomach can be divided with a 90-mm linear stapler with 4.8-mm staples. The jejunum is brought up in an antecolic fashion to the greater curve side of the stomach. Traction sutures of 4-0 silk are placed in the antimesenteric side of the jejunum and on the posterior surface of the stomach, approximately 2 cm proximal to the gastric staple line. (Figure 15-21) A small jejunotomy and gastrotomy are created at the same level with the electrocautery just inferior to the stay sutures. The anvil of the 45-mm linear cutter is placed in the jejunum and the stapling fork placed in the gastric lumen. The stapler is closed, ensuring that no tissue is incorporated in the staple closure. There should be 2 cm of gastric wall between the gastric staple line and the linear cutter, and the tissue of the gastric wall and jejunum should be approximated. (Figure 15-22) The stapler is fired and removed. The staple line is inspected internally by using a ring clamp. The common enterotomy is grasped with two Allis clamps and closed with a linear stapler. The stapler must include a full-thickness bite of the entire opening to ensure adequate closure. The staple lines can be inverted with an interrupted layer of Lembert stitches, but this is not necessary.

♦ If a gastrojejunal, or Billroth II, anastomosis is to be performed, the duodenal stump must be closed. It has been said that "if one can close the duodenum, one can anastomose to it." In the hands of expert gastric surgeons this is probably true; however, with fewer gastric resections being performed, the experience level has diminished drastically, and the surgeon should select the best anastomosis for the situation given his or her comfort level. The healthy, pliable duodenal stump is best closed in two layers. A Connell stitch is used to invert the mucosa of the duodenum. (Figure 15-23ABC) Sutures of 4-0 polyglactin are run from each end of the duodenal opening and secured to one another in the middle. A second interrupted layer of 4-0 silk or polyglactin suture is placed in a Lembert fashion. If the duodenum is not adequately pliable, the second seromuscular layer of stitches should be omitted. A linear stapler may be used as well to close the healthy duodenal stump. A 55-mm stapler with a 3.5-mm or 4.8-mm staple height cartridge should be used. However, if the duodenal wall is diseased enough to think that sutures will not hold, stapling will fail also.

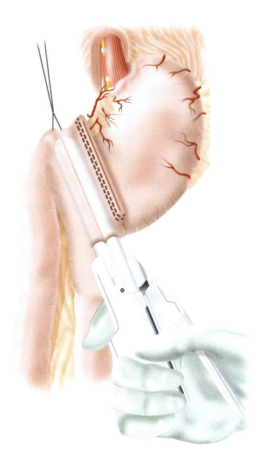

Figure 15-21

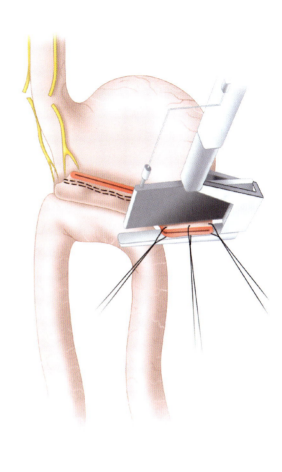

Figure 15-22

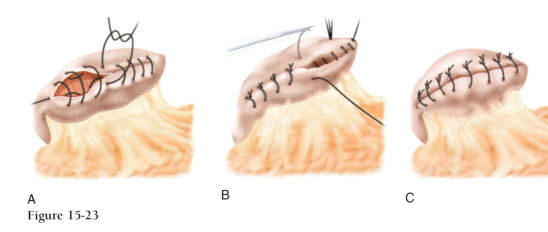

A

B

C

Figure 15-23

- The difficult duodenal stump requires the surgeon to have a few options for closure. When the posterior duodenal wall contains a penetrating ulcer or it is too scarred to free up, the pliable anterior wall of the duodenum is used to close the defect. This technique requires a Kocher maneuver to gain mobility of the duodenum. The Nissen-Cooper technique of duodenal closure consists of two layers of interrupted Lembert stitches to accomplish closure. The first layer of sutures uses 4-0 silk or polyglactin suture to attach the anterior wall of the duodenum to the distal lip of the ulcer. A second layer of Lembert sutures inverts the first suture line by securing the pliable anterior duodenal wall to the proximal ulcer edge and pancreatic capsule. (Figure 15-24AB) Another technique for closure in more experienced hands is to perform a gastroduodenostomy to incorporate duodenal closure. A modification of the usual Billroth I reconstruction is made. The posterior wall of the duodenum, which is in the region of the ulcer crater, is sewn to the stomach with a single layer of 4-0 silk or polyglactin sutures. The bites should include the stomach, underlying fibrosed pancreas, and distal lip of the ulcer crater and duodenum. The knot is tied on the inside of the lumen. (Figure 15-25)

3. Closing

- The position of the nasogastric tube is confirmed intraoperatively. The tip of the tube should be in the body of the stomach and not in the area of the suture line.
- Once hemostasis is confirmed, the incision is closed with running absorbable, monofilamented sutures.
- Drains are not typically left in the operative field unless there was a difficult duodenal stump. In this situation, a closed suction drain is left in the vicinity of the duodenal closure. Omentum should be placed between the drain tip and the suture line.

Step 4: Postoperative Care

- Initially, the patient's hydration status must be maintained with intravenous fluids. A urinary catheter, with output recorded every shift, helps guide resuscitation. The nasogastric tube is connected to low, intermittent suction and output recorded each shift. The tube should be flushed with small amounts of saline to ensure patency of the drain and prevent gastric distention. Excessive losses from the nasogastric tube should be replaced.
- Electrolytes should be checked daily as long as the patient is receiving intravenous fluids. Once diet is resumed, they should be monitored every 2 to 3 days.
- The patient's weight should be recorded daily. Dietary instructions include frequent, small meals and avoidance of concentrated carbohydrates. Foods restricted preoperatively should be resumed one at a time. Ultimately, the only dietary restrictions are the ones imposed by individual intolerance.
- Long-term follow-up is required to determine the success of the operation. A return to an unlimited diet with maintenance of ideal body weight and absence of chronic gastrointestinal complaints should be the goals.

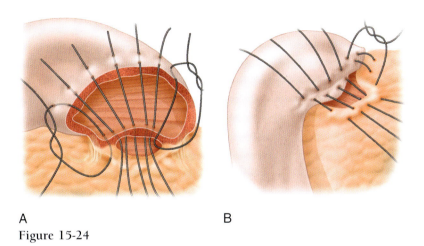

A   B

Figure 15-24

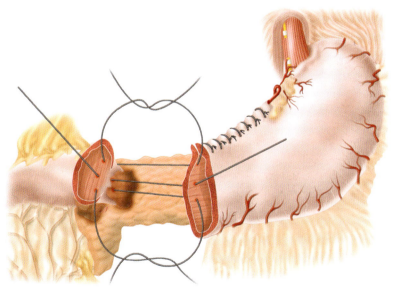

Figure 15-25

Step 5: Pearls and Pitfalls

- When initially assessing the quality of the duodenum to determine feasibility of antrectomy, a small incision in the anterior duodenum may be made to inspect the ulcer pathology. When in doubt, it is always preferable to perform a vagotomy and drainage procedure incorporating the duodenotomy, rather than risk a resection with the possibility of a duodenal leakage or pancreatitis.
- If division of the stomach is performed using a linear stapler, always ensure that the nasogastric tube has been pulled back into the esophagus. Dividing the tube with the stapler may not be recognized at the time, and it will require another laparotomy to remove.
- For a difficult duodenal stump, a lateral catheter duodenostomy is a nice adjunct to protect the closure. Before closure of the stump, a right-angled clamp is passed through the lumen and pressed against the lateral wall of the ascending duodenum. A tiny duodenotomy is made in the lateral ascending wall of the duodenum. A 14-French Foley catheter is passed to the right-angled clamp and brought into the lumen. The catheter is sewn in place with a 4-0 polyglactin purse string suture. The catheter is brought out through a stab wound in the abdominal wall leaving adequate slack to allow for abdominal distention. The catheter is placed to low suction until flatus returns. It can then be placed to gravity drainage and removed on postoperative day 8.

References

1. Aoki T: Current status of and problems in the treatment of gastric and duodenal ulcer disease: introduction. *World J Surg* 2000; 24:249.
2. Dempsey D, Ashley S, Mercer DW, et al. Peptic ulcer surgery in the H. pylori era: indications for operation. *Contemp Surg* 2001; 57:433-441.
3. Herrington JL. Vagotomy-antrectomy: how I do it. Acta Chi Scand Suppl 1992; 72:335,.
4. Mercer DW, Robinson EK: Stomach. In: Townsend CM, Jr., ed. *Sabiston textbook of surgery: the biological basis of modern surgical practice.* 17th ed. Philadelphia: Saunders Elsevier; 2004.
5. Nyhus LM: Selective vagotomy, antrectomy, and gastroduodenostomy for the treatment of duodenal ulcer. In: Nyhus LM, Baker RJ, eds. *Mastery of surgery.* 2nd ed. Boston: Little, Brown, and Co.; 1992.
6. Scott-Connor CEH. Gastrectomy (antrectomy) for peptic ulcer: surgical legacy technique. In: Scott-Connor CEH, ed. *Chassin's operative strategy in general surgery.* 3rd ed. New York: Springer; Inc., 2002.

CHAPTER 16

SURGICAL TREATMENT OF POSTGASTRECTOMY SYNDROMES

Alfredo M. Carbonell, DO, FACS, FACOS

Step 1: Surgical Anatomy

- ◆ Due to the multiplicity of gastric operations performed both for benign and malignant diseases, it is imperative that the reoperative surgeon obtain and review all prior operative reports relating to the index gastric procedures. Prior knowledge and understanding of the patient's anatomy and symptoms will allow the surgeon to accurately decide which remedial operation is appropriate for which postgastrectomy syndrome.

Step 2: Preoperative Considerations

- ◆ Preoperative endoscopy, contrast upper gastrointestinal radiographs, and biliary nuclear scans can all aid the surgeon in making the appropriate diagnosis of a postgastrectomy syndrome.

Step 3: Operative Steps

1. Dumping

- ◆ Classic early dumping, characterized by rapid postprandial weakness, dizziness, palpitations, diaphoresis, abdominal cramping, and explosive diarrhea, occurs as a result of increased gastric emptying after pyloroplasty or antrectomy.

- ◆ Roux-en-Y diversion after a previous complete vagal denervation will significantly delay gastric emptying and reverse the dumping syndrome, which is why it is the remedial surgery of choice for this ailment.
  - ▲ Conversion prior truncal vagotomy and pyloroplasty to 50 cm Roux-en-Y anastomosis. (Figure 16-1A)
  - ▲ Conversion truncal vagotomy and antrectomy (Billroth I) to 50 cm Roux-en-Y anastomosis. (Figure 16-1B)
  - ▲ Conversion truncal vagotomy and antrectomy (Billroth II) to 50 cm Roux-en-Y anastomosis. (Figure 16-1C)

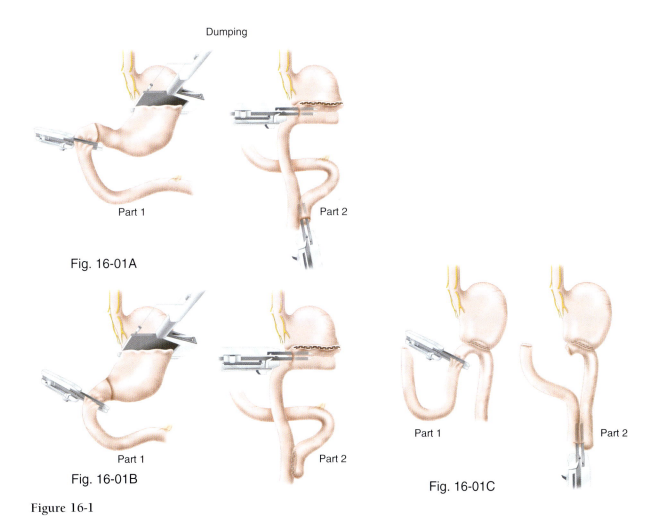

Dumping

Part 1

Part 2

Fig. 16-01A

Part 1

Part 2

Fig. 16-01B

Part 1

Part 2

Fig. 16-01C

Figure 16-1

2. Gastroparesis

- Chronic gastroparesis can present with nausea, vomiting, abdominal pain, postprandial bloating, and bezoar formation.
- The remedial operation should be predicated on the need to remove a portion of the atonic stomach.
- A previous truncal vagotomy with pyloroplasty will mandate a 50% gastrectomy with a Billroth II reconstruction. The addition of a Braun enteroenterostomy 25 cm distal to the Billroth II gastrojejunostomy will divert a major portion of bile from the stomach, preventing bile reflux gastritis. (Figure 16-2A).
- A previous antrectomy requires a subtotal gastrectomy with Bilroth II reconstruction. If a Roux-en-Y reconstruction is planned then a near total gastrectomy should be performed.
- Conversion of a truncal vagotomy and antrectomy (Billroth I or II) to a subtotal gastrectomy (>25%) with a Billroth II reconstruction and a Braun enteroenterostomy (Figure 16-2B) or near total gastrectomy (<25%) gastrectomy with Roux-en-Y reconstruction (Figure 16-2C).

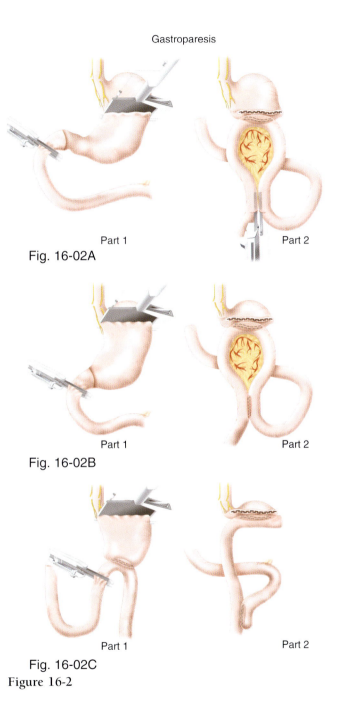

Gastroparesis

Part 1   Part 2

Fig. 16-02A

Part 1   Part 2

Fig. 16-02B

Part 1   Part 2

Fig. 16-02C

Figure 16-2

3. Alkaline Reflux

- Alkaline reflux, although typically a diagnosis of exclusion, presents with severe burning and upper abdominal pain. Endoscopic findings of gastritis and a quantitative radionuclide biliary scan for enterogastric reflux can aid in the diagnosis.
- The remedial operation mandates enough of a gastric resection to prevent postsurgical gastric atony. In addition, a Roux-en-Y reconstruction will allow for complete biliary diversion.
- Conversion of a truncal vagotomy and pyloroplasty to a hemigastrectomy with Roux-en-Y. (Figure 16-3A)
- Conversion of a truncal vagotomy and antrectomy (Billroth I) to a hemigastrectomy with Roux-en-Y. (Figure 16-3B)
- Conversion of a truncal vagotomy and antrectomy (Billroth II) to a subtotal gastrectomy with Roux-en-Y. (Figure 16-3C)

Alkaline Reflux

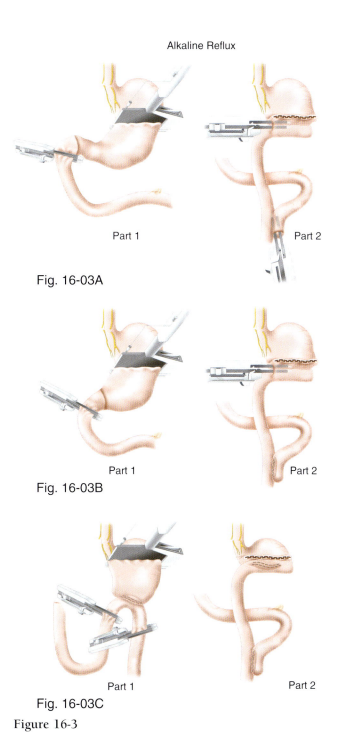

Part 1

Part 2

Fig. 16-03A

Part 1

Part 2

Fig. 16-03B

Part 1

Part 2

Fig. 16-03C

Figure 16-3

4. Roux Stasis Syndrome

- ◆ Roux stasis is a subtle finding that mimics gastroparesis. In fact, most patients with this syndrome have both an atonic stomach and delayed emptying of the Roux limb.
- ◆ The remedial operation should, at minimum, address the gastric atony by gastric resection, particularly if there has been a previous antrectomy or hemigastrectomy. If the patient has already had a subtotal gastrectomy, consideration can be given to reversal of the Roux-en-Y.
- ◆ Conversion of an antrectomy with Roux-en-Y to a subtotal gastrectomy with Roux-en-Y. (Figure 16-4A)
- ◆ Conversion of an antrectomy with Roux-en-Y to a subtotal gastrectomy and reversal of the Roux-en-Y anastomosis to a Billroth II-type reconstruction with a Braun enteroenterostomy. (Figure 16-4B)

5. Afferent or Efferent Loop Syndrome

- ◆ Treatment of this syndrome requires revision or resection of the previous anastomotic stricture. A Billroth II with Braun enteroenterostomy will prevent future alkaline gastric reflux.
- ◆ Revise the gastrojejunostomy staple line. (Figure 16-5A)
- ◆ Resect and reconstruct Billroth II with Braun enteroenterostomy. (Figure 16-5B)

References

1. Ritchie WP, Jr. Alkaline reflux gastritis. *Gastroenterol Clin North Am* 1994; 23(2):281-294.
2. Vogel SB. Surgery for postgastrectomy syndromes. In: Nyhus LM, Baker RJ, Fischer JE, eds. *Mastery of surgery.* Vol. 1. Boston: Little, Brown and Company; 1997.
3. Vogel SB, Drane WE, Woodward ER. Clinical and radionuclide evaluation of bile diversion by Braun enteroenterostomy: prevention and treatment of alkaline reflux gastritis. An alternative to Roux-en-Y diversion. *Ann Surg* 1994; 219(5):458-465; discussion 465-466.
4. Vogel SB, Hocking MP, Woodward ER. Clinical and radionuclide evaluation of Roux-Y diversion for postgastrectomy dumping. *Am J Surg* 1988; 155(1):57-62.
5. Woodward ER, Hocking MP. Postgastrectomy syndromes. *Surg Clin North Am* 1987; 67(3):509-520.

Roux Stasis Syndrome

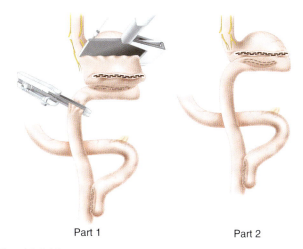

Part 1   Part 2

Fig. 16-04A

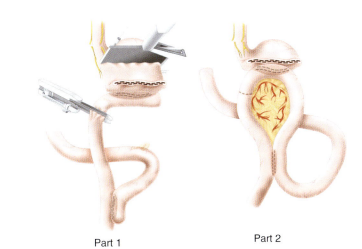

Part 1   Part 2

Fig. 16-04B

Figure 16-4

Afferent or Efferent Loop Syndrome

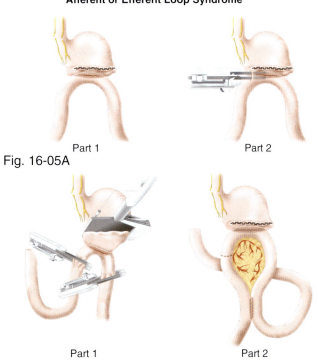

Part 1   Part 2

Fig. 16-05A

Part 1   Part 2

Fig. 16-05B

Figure 16-5

CHAPTER 17

LAPAROSCOPIC GASTRIC ULCER SURGERY

William S. Cobb IV, MD

Step 1: Surgical Anatomy

- Division of the vagus nerves is an important part of any operation whose goal is to control gastric acid secretion. The left vagus nerve that crosses anteriorly at the distal esophagus and the right vagus branch that crosses posteriorly can be interrupted intraabdominally by one of three main operations. A truncal vagotomy consists of the two trunks being divided approximately 5 cm cephalad from the gastroesophageal junction. A selective vagotomy involves division of the vagal branches distal to the celiac (posterior) and hepatic (anterior) branches. This operation is not commonly performed. A highly selective, or parietal cell, vagotomy results in denervation of only the proximal two thirds of the stomach by dividing the anterior and posterior nerves of Latarjet.

Step 2: Preoperative Considerations

- With the improved medical agents to control gastric acid and the increased understanding of the role of *H. pylori* infection, few patients are candidates for surgical intervention for gastric and duodenal ulcer disease. More often, surgical therapy is relegated to those patients with severe and emergent complications of ulcer disease. The recent advances in video optics and instruments coupled with the growing number of laparoscopic surgeons comfortable with procedures on the foregut, such as fundoplications and Roux-en-Y gastrojejunostomies, have led to the application of minimally invasive techniques for ulcer disease.
- A minimally invasive approach may potentially reduce the immediate postoperative morbidity following surgery for ulcer disease. The indications for laparoscopic therapy for ulcer disease remain the same as for open surgery: failure of medical therapy, and obstruction, perforation, and concern for malignancy. Common minimally invasive antiulcer procedures include truncal vagotomy and antrectomy with either Billroth I or Billroth II reconstruction; vagotomy and pyloroplasty; and parietal cell vagotomy. Several series, largely from Europe, report good results with ulcer recurrence using a posterior truncal vagotomy combined with either an anterior seromyotomy or anterior linear gastrectomy. For patients with gastric outlet obstruction, a laparoscopic truncal vagotomy with pyloroplasty, and vagotomy with antrectomy are both

valid surgical options. If a perforation occurs, a laparoscopic omental patch with simple closure, followed by peritoneal lavage, is suitable most of the time. A more definitive antiulcer procedure may be performed if there is minimal contamination and the condition of the patient allows it.

- Laparoscopy requires pneumoperitoneum, so the acutely ill or septic patient may not tolerate increased intraabdominal pressure and would not be a candidate for a laparoscopic approach. Relative contraindications to a laparoscopic approach include an acutely bleeding ulcer and the difficult duodenal stump.
- The preoperative evaluation of the ulcer patient for laparoscopy is similar to that for open gastric procedures. Patients with acute gastroduodenal perforations must be hemodynamically stable to tolerate pneumoperitoneum. Chronically ill patients with ulcer disease should have their nutritional status optimized.

Step 3: Operative Steps

1. Incision

- Trocar placement mimics that of most laparoscopic foregut procedures. The patient is placed in the lithotomy position with the use of stirrups or, preferably, a split-leg table. (Figure 17-1)
- All 5-mm trocars are suitable if no specimens are to be retrieved and no staplers are to be used. The curved suture needle can be bent to resemble a ski needle to fit through the 5-mm trocar.

2. Dissection

Laparoscopic closure of gastroduodenal perforation
- Different techniques have been described for laparoscopic treatment of a perforated peptic ulcer. Following the principle of conventional open repair, ulcer closure may be performed by simple or running suture techniques incorporating omental patches. (Figure 17-2)
- Laparoscopic guided techniques for creating plugs of omentum of the ligamentum teres hepatis have been described. Sutureless techniques including plugs of gelatin sponges or fibrin glue have been used but are associated with higher leak rates, particularly if the perforation is larger than 5 mm in diameter. A simple suture technique incorporating an omental patch based on Graham's closure and not using any additional foreign bodies is preferable.
- The peritoneal cavity is then copiously irrigated with several liters of warm normal saline. All four quadrants and especially the pelvic cavity should be rinsed until the effluent is clear. Tilting the patient from side to side and using Trendelenburg and reverse Trendelenburg positions assist with irrigation.

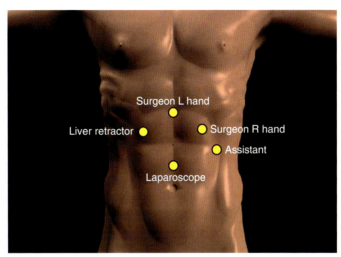

Figure 17-1

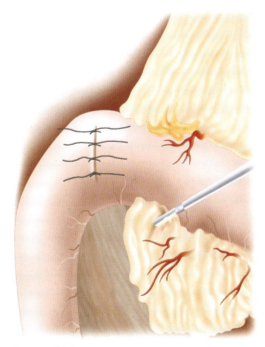

Figure 17-2

3. Laparoscopic Highly Selective Vagotomy

♦ The peritoneal cavity is accessed safely just above the umbilicus, approximately 12 cm from the xiphoid process. An open cut-down technique or optical trocar may be used to gain entry. The additional 5-mm trocars are placed as shown in Figure 17-1. A liver retractor is brought in through the right upper quadrant trocar and secured with a stationary side-rail mounted arm.

♦ The planned extent of the vagotomy is marked with sutures. A stitch is placed just to the left of the anterior vagus nerve where it emerges from under the peritoneum at the gastroesophageal junction. A second stitch marks the lower limit of the planned vagotomy, usually at the level of the first branch of the crow's foot. (Figure 17-3)

♦ The direction of dissection is from caudad to cephalad. Maintaining hemostasis is paramount to prevent blood staining of the tissues and hematoma formation, which can obscure identification of the neurovascular pedicles. The ultrasonic shears work nicely and reduce thermal spread to surrounding tissue. Hemoclips are used for larger vessels. All anterior leaflet vessels are divided from the crow's foot to the angle of His. (Figure 17-4)

♦ The division of the posterior leaflet is continued by entering the lesser sac. The greater curvature of the stomach is elevated, and the omentum divided with ultrasonic shears to open the lesser sac. The posterior aspect of the stomach is then regrasped to expose the posterior crow's foot. The posterior vagus nerve is seen crossing an arcade of vessels at this point. (Figure 17-5) The vessel is divided with clips. A Penrose drain is looped around the distal stomach at the crow's foot to provide downward traction. (Figure 17-6) Dissection proceeds toward the gastroesophageal junction. The free edge of the lesser omentum is divided with ultrasonic shears separating it from the lesser curve of the stomach.

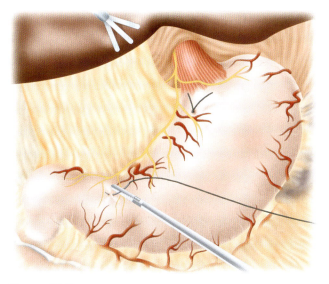

Figure 17-3

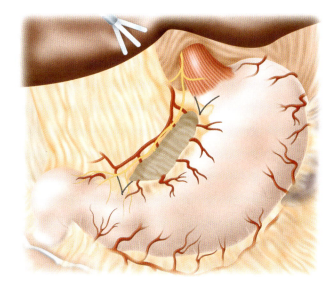

Figure 17-4

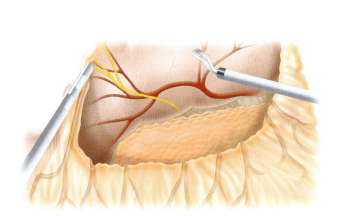

Figure 17-5

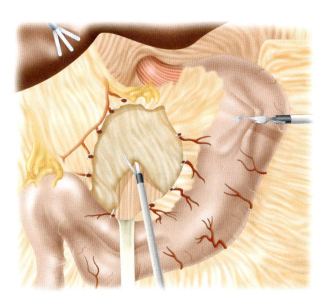

Figure 17-6

◆ The distal 5 cm of the esophagus should be cleared of any vagal branches. The dissection extends from the lowermost esophagus to the partially divided crow's foot. (Figure 17-7)

4. Laparoscopic Truncal Vagotomy and Pyloroplasty

◆ Truncal vagotomy provides treatment of refractory ulcer disease with reduced rates of recurrence. Denervation of the vagal fibers to the distal stomach results in altered antral motility, and therefore, an emptying procedure is required. A Heineke-Mikulicz pyloroplasty is commonly used.

◆ Dissection begins at the esophageal hiatus. The left lobe of the liver is elevated, exposing the pars flaccida of the lesser omentum, which is incised with the ultrasonic shears. The plane between the right crus and the esophagus is bluntly developed. Only a thin layer of loose areolar tissue separates the phrenoesophageal ligament from the esophagus. Care should be taken not to damage the fascia overlying the crus. If the muscle fibers of the crus are visible, dissection is in the wrong plane.

◆ Dissection along the crus continues inferiorly toward the junction of the crural fibers. When the left crus is seen joining its right counterpart, a plane is bluntly developed anterior to the crura. This dissection essentially creates a retroesophageal window. A Penrose drain cut to 18 cm is passed through this window and used for retraction.

◆ The esophagus is circumferentially mobilized into the mediastinum. Again, this is largely performed bluntly; however, the ultrasonic shears may be needed to control small vessels. If significant bleeding occurs, the dissection plane is too close to the esophagus.

◆ The anterior vagus nerve is visualized passing from left to right obliquely on the anterior surface of the esophagus. Placing caudal retraction on the esophagus with a Penrose drain places tension on the nerve and makes it easier to identify. (Figure 17-8) Two Maryland dissectors allow for elevation of the nerve while spreading the surrounding tissue deep to it. The nerve is freed from the longitudinal fibers of the esophagus for approximately 4 to 5 cm and divided between clips. A specimen is sent to pathology for confirmation.

◆ The posterior vagus is exposed by retracting the esophagus toward the patient's left shoulder. (Figure 17-9) It is mobilized off the esophagus in a similar fashion as described for the anterior branch.

◆ A Heineke-Mikulicz pyloroplasty is performed as described in Chapter 12. The pyloric vein of Mayo provides a distal landmark. The ultrasonic shears create a gastrostomy that is extended longitudinally onto the duodenum. The opening is closed transversely with interrupted 2-0 silk or polyglactin sutures. A linear stapler may be utilized to close the gastrotomy as well.

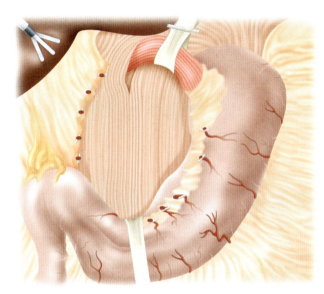

Figure 17-7

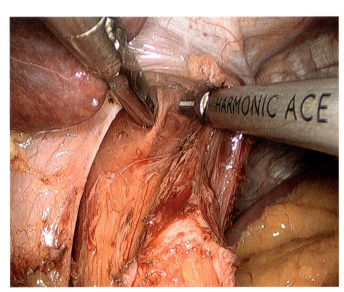

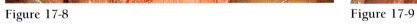

Figure 17-8

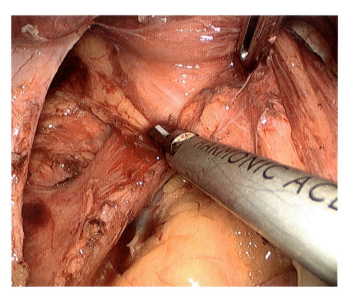

Figure 17-9

5. Closing

◆ The fascia at trocar sites greater than 5 mm is closed with the fascial closure device and 0 polyglactin suture. The skin is closed with 4-0 poliglecaprone 25, and surgical glue is applied to the skin closure.

Step 4: Postoperative Care

◆ Following perforations, a nasogastric tube is left postoperatively for decompression. The degree of adynamic ileus depends on the amount of contamination. The patient's diet is advanced slowly, starting with clear liquids as bowel function returns. Broad-spectrum antibiotics are continued postoperatively in cases with a lot of contamination.

◆ The postoperative course following elective antiulcer procedures is usually uneventful. A nasogastric tube is not usually required if there have been no perforations. The diet may be resumed starting with clear liquids the first postoperative morning.

Step 5: Pearls and Pitfalls

◆ The benefits of a laparoscopic approach to perforated gastroduodenal ulcers are several-fold. The minimally invasive technique reduces the trauma of a laparotomy in a patient population that many times is high risk. Laparoscopy can help confirm or refute the diagnosis, and if the perforation is already sealed off by omentum, some authors have advocated leaving the omentum intact and laparoscopically performing peritoneal lavage.

References

1. Casas AT, Gadacz TR. Laparoscopic management of peptic ulcer disease. *Surg Clin North Am* 1996; 76:515-522.
2. Dallemagne B, Weerts JM, Jehaes C, et al. Laparoscopic highly selective vagotomy. *Br J Surg* 1994; 81:554-556.
3. Katkhouda N, Waldrup D, Campos G, et al. An improved technique for laparoscopic highly selective vagotomy using harmonic shears. *Surg Endosc* 1998; 12:1051-1054.

CHAPTER 18

SUBTOTAL GASTRECTOMY: BILLROTH I AND II

Julian A. Kim, MD, FACS

Step 1: Surgical Anatomy

- The arterial blood supply to the stomach is rich and comes from multiple sources. These include the left gastric artery (branch of the celiac axis), right gastric artery (branch of the hepatic artery), and right and left gastroepiploic arteries, which form an arcade along the greater curvature and short gastric arteries from the superior pole of the spleen that supply the cardia. In general, maintenance of the short gastric arteries is enough to provide adequate arterial blood supply to the gastric remnant during subtotal gastrectomy.

- Lymph node basins in which gastric cancer can commonly spread can be divided into various regions based upon their proximity to the primary tumor. Perigastric lymph nodes and those near the left gastric artery and celiac axis are considered first-echelon nodal basins. Lymph nodes along the common hepatic artery, porta hepatis, aorta, and peripancreatic and perisplenic left renal hilum are considered second-echelon nodal basins and can be resected with increased morbidity and debatable improvements in overall survival.

- Cancers of the stomach can be in proximity or directly invade the distal esophagus, diaphragmatic hiatus or crura, pericardium, spleen, celiac axis, pancreas, adrenal gland, and left kidney. They can also frequently metastasize to the omentum, peritoneum, and liver. Gastric cancers that are best treated by subtotal gastrectomy are those that involve the antrum or fundus; tumors of the proximal stomach and cardia are best served by total gastrectomy or esophagogastrectomy.

Step 2: Preoperative Considerations

- It is critically important to properly stage any patient who is being considered for subtotal gastrectomy for cancer prior to any operative intervention. Patients with locally advanced tumors that are directly invading surrounding structures such as the main celiac trunk, diaphragmatic hiatus, or pericardium, as well as those patients who present with metastases to liver or lung may be best served with some combination of systemic therapy and radiation, depending upon whether they have symptoms of bleeding or obstruction. In general these advanced tumors have a low chance of cure and any surgical attempts are oriented towards palliation.

▲ Upper endoscopy and endoscopic ultrasound can be useful in determining the location and extent of disease spread within the gastric wall, as well as providing a method of diagnosis via endoscopic biopsy.

▲ Submucosal tumors should be sent for CD117 immunostaining to determine whether a gastrointestinal stromal tumor is present. These tumors, if small and localized, can sometimes be resected via wedge resection, and subtotal gastrectomy can be avoided.

▲ Biopsies of mucosal tumors that demonstrate a diffuse, infiltrative signet ring cell histology may be best served with total gastrectomy, particularly if the mucosal ulcerations extend over a broad surface towards the proximal stomach.

▲ Anesthesia considerations are similar to any major abdominal surgical procedure. The anesthesia team should be aware of the need for possible insertion and manipulation of a nasogastric tube, as well as the possibility of intraoperative endoscopy.

▲ Patient instructions and consent are also important for success. Patients should be aware of prolonged hospitalization, which could be related to possible complications from anastomotic leaks or intraabdominal abscesses. The patient will likely lose up to 10% to 20% of their body weight and may not regain it after the surgery. They may also require prolonged enteral nutritional supplements via jejunostomy feedings, and they should be made aware of this possibility.

Step 3: Operative Steps

♦ In general, it is reasonable to perform intraoperative upper endoscopy and diagnostic laparoscopy to help plan surgical resection. Those patients with unsuspected metastatic disease to the peritoneum or liver may be best served with feeding jejunostomy if the patient has limited symptoms. The use of self-retaining retractor systems will facilitate exposure and ease of operation.

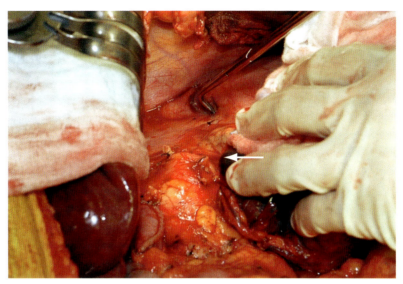

Figure 18-1. Dissection along the lesser curvature of the stomach is accomplished with retraction of the stomach to the patient's left. The left lateral segment of the liver is retracted to the right. Incision of the lesser omentum exposes the caudate lobe of the liver, right crus of diaphragm, abdominal aorta and celiac axis (arrow). Tumor involving the celiac axis may restrict control of the left gastric artery and can be a relative contraindication to subtotal gastrectomy.

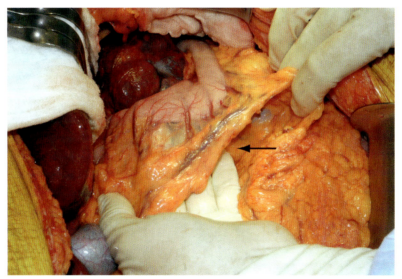

Figure 18-2. The left gastroepiploic artery arises from the gastroduodenal artery and joins the right gastroepiploic artery to supply the greater curvature of the stomach. Dissection along the gastroepiploic vessels detaches the greater omentum from the stomach and allows access to the posterior wall of the stomach, body and tail of the pancreas and assessment of the celiac axis to determine resectability prior to division of the left and right gastric arteries.

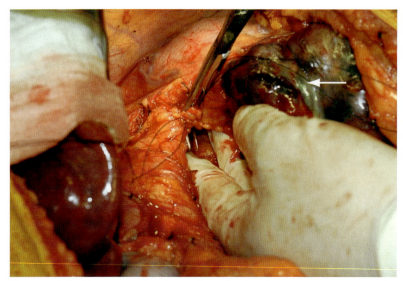

Figure 18-3. Tumor-involved lymph nodes (in this case metastatic melanoma) must be cleared from the origin of the left gastric artery prior to ligation. It is sometimes helpful to ligate the proximal left gastric artery prior to extensive manipulation to ensure proximal arterial control. The left gastric artery is a thin-walled visceral artery and should be suture-ligated or oversewn. Loss of control of the left gastric artery stump can lead to inadvertent injury to the celiac axis or abdominal aorta.

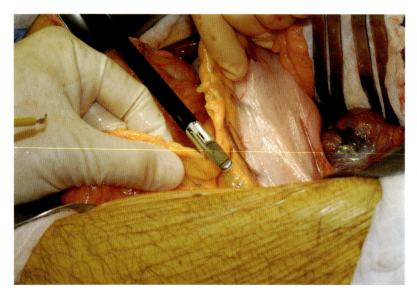

Figure 18-4. If the omentum is not being removed, the greater curvature of the stomach can be released from the omentum by either ligatures or an automated device. Dissection should be carried outside of the gastroepiploic vessels in order to include the perigastric lymph nodes. This dissection should stop before encountering the short gastric vessels for subtotal gastrectomy, particularly if the left gastric artery has been divided.

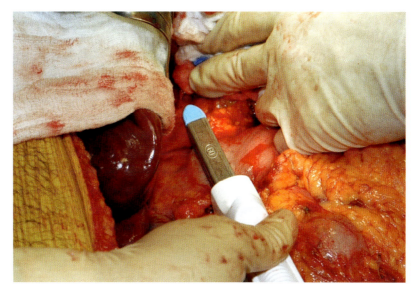

Figure 18-5. After the arterial supply has been divided, the proximal duodenal bulb is divided immediately distal to the pylorus. The pyloric vein can be used as a landmark if the anatomy is difficult. The duodenal bulb should then be oversewn with interrrupted or continous suture in order to avoid stump "blowout". A drain may be placed at the duodenal stump to alert to bilious leakage prior to the patient exhibiting signs of sepsis.

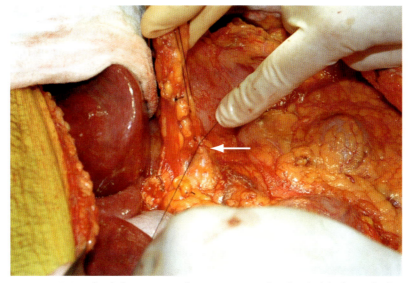

Figure 18-6. The left gastroepiploic artery can be divided before of after division of the duodenal bulb. This artery can be identified by following the gastroepiploic arcade along the greater curvature toward the pylorus. The origin of the left gastroepiploic artery (arrow) is in close proximity to the anterior surface of the pancreas and care must be taken not to disrupt the pancreatic gland capsule. Tumors of the antrum may involve the pancreas by direct extension and should be managed by en bloc distal or subtotal pancreatectomy.

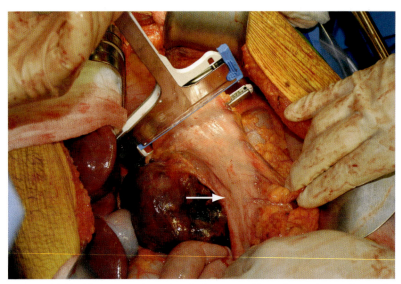

Figure 18-7. The stomach is divided proximally at least 5 cm above the gastric tumor. If a 5 cm margin cannot be achieved, total gastrectomy should be considered. The stomach is divided proximal to the incisura angularis (arrow). If a stapling device is used, care should be taken to make sure that the nasogastric tube or any intragastric devices have been removed prior to firing the stapler. There is no need to mobilize the esophagus or perform a total vagotomy as the acid secreting portion of the stomach is being removed.

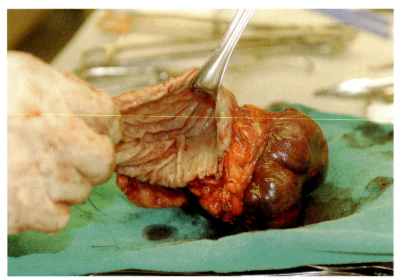

Figure 18-8. It is a good idea to open the proximal suture line of the specimen to determine whether a gross tumor resection has been achieved. If additional resection needs to be performed it can be done before the roux-en-y gastrojejunostomy. In general Billroth I and II reconstruction following subtotal gastrectomy can lead to significant bile reflux gastritis.

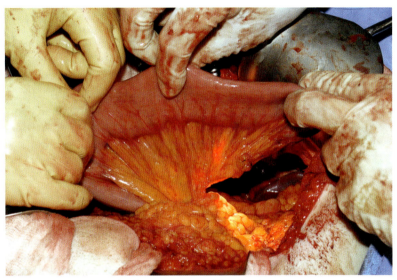

Figure 18-9. A roux limb is constructed by dividing the proximal jejunum and mesentery. The roux limb can be advanced through a window in the transverse mesocolon to the left of the middle colic artery to the level of the proximal stomach. A two-layer anastamosis is performed and a naso-gastric tube passed through the anastamosis. The roux limb should be sutured to the mesocolic window and the defect closed in order to avoid an internal hernia. The gastrojejunal anastomosis technique is covered in previous chapters.

Step 4: Postoperative Care

- As with any upper abdominal surgery, early mobilization of the patient and aggressive pulmonary toilet should be instituted. Adequate pain control via epidural catheter, subcutaneous local anesthesia catheter, or patient-controlled anesthestic devices will assist in recovery.
  - ▲ Early intestinal feedings and nutritional support are preferred even after the patient starts oral feedings. It is likely that patients will have to alter their eating habits with small frequent meals following subtotal gastrectomy.
  - ▲ Upper gastrointestinal studies to check for anastomotic integrity are not essential but can be helpful, particularly if patients exhibit unexpected fever, abdominal pain, flank pain, or shoulder pain in the early postoperative period.

Step 5: Pearls and Pitfalls

- It is critically important to accurately stage the tumor preoperatively to determine whether the resection can be done from a strictly abdominal approach.
- En bloc resection of associated organs (distal pancreatectomy, resection of colonic mesentery) can be performed if the tumor directly invades these structures but will result in increased surgical morbidity.
- In general, splenic preservation is preferred unless the tumor directly invades the spleen.
- It is ok to resect the left gastric artery as long as the short gastric arteries are left intact.

CHAPTER 19

TOTAL GASTRECTOMY

Julian A. Kim, MD, FACS

Step 1: Surgical Anatomy

- The arterial blood supply to the stomach was covered in Chapter 18. The blood supply for the distal esophagus is derived from perforating arterial branches from the aorta. Extensive mobilization of the distal esophagus may interrupt these arteries and compromise the arterial blood supply.
- The vagus nerves run parallel to the distal esophagus. The right vagus nerve trunk can be spared during esophageal transaction in order to preserve branches to the gallbladder.

Step 2: Preoperative Considerations

- In patients who are scheduled for total gastrectomy, the proximal extent of disease is critical to determine whether a distal esophagectomy should be performed. Preoperative endoscopy images should be carefully reviewed, including a phone conversation with the referring gastroenterologist or surgeon. Imaging studies such as CT scans and PETs may be helpful in identifying extent of metastases as well.
- Tumors of the gastroesophageal junction usually require distal esophagectomy, which can be performed via a left thoracoabdominal, abdominal right thoracic (Ivor Lewis), or transhiatal approach. Patients who present with gastroesophageal junction tumors should be carefully assessed prior to scheduling for any surgical procedure.
- Anesthesiologists should be aware of the possible need for extension of incisions into the thoracic cavities. In the event that this is necessary, a dual lumen endotracheal tube and single lung ventilation may be necessary during a portion of the operative procedure.

Step 3: Operative Steps

- ◆ Intraoperative endoscopy and diagnostic laparoscopy may be helpful in confirming the extent of disease. The right and left chest should be prepped in the operative field in case an extension of the incision is necessary. The proximal stomach and distal esophagus can be accessed via midline laparotomy or bilateral subcostal incisions with a vertical extension. Self-retaining retractors are again helpful in providing exposure.

Step 4: Postoperative Care

- ◆ As with any upper abdominal surgery, early mobilization of the patient and agressive pulmonary toilet should be instituted. Adequate pain control via epidural catheter, subcutaneous local anesthesia catheter, or patient-controlled anesthestic devices will assist in recovery.
  - ▲ Early intestinal feedings and nutritional support are preferred even after the patient starts oral feedings. It is likely that patients will have to alter their eating habits with small frequent meals following subtotal gastrectomy.
  - ▲ Upper gastrointestinal studies to check for anastomotic integrity are not essential but can be helpful, particularly if patients exhibit unexpected fever, abdominal pain, flank pain, or shoulder pain in the early postoperative period.

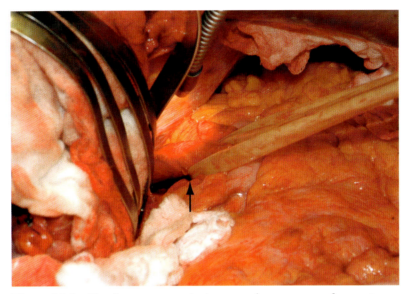

Figure 19-1. The first manuver during a total gastrectomy for carcinoma is to assess the proximal extent of disease. The left lateral segment of the liver is retracted to the right and the gastrophrenic ligament is incised. The esophagus is encircled with a Penrose drain (arrow) and 5-6 cm of esophagus is mobilized into the abdomen. If there is palpable evidence of disease in the distal esophagus, an intra-operative EGD should be performed to ensure that resection can be performed from within the abdomen with clear margins.

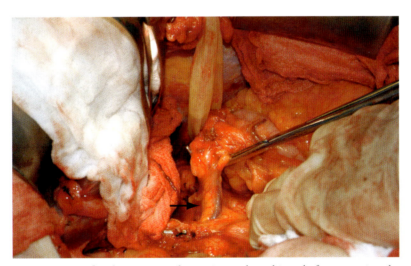

Figure 19-2. If a clear proximal margin can be achieved after assessing the distal esophagus, the celiac axis is then assessed to ensure resectability (arrow). The celiac lymphadenectomy can be extended proximally along the abdominal aorta to the right crus of the diaphragm. The dissection is continued to the level of the Penrose drain which is encircling the esophagus to completely mobilize the lesser curvature of the stomach.

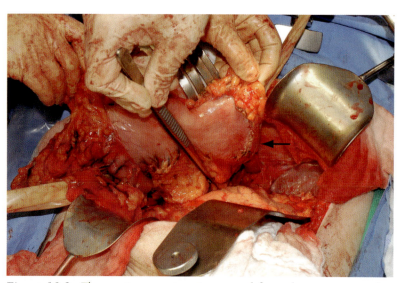

Figure 19-3. The greater omentum is resected from the transverse colon starting from the hepatic flexure and extending to the splenic flexure. The dissection is continued along the greater curvature of the stomach to the level of the short gastric arteries (arrow). These arteries are carefully ligated or divided using an automated device. Splenectomy is not necessary unless the tumor directly invades into the spleen. The dissection is then carried along the cardia and the left crus of the diaphragm to the Penrose drain which is encircling the esophagus to complete the greater curvature mobilization.

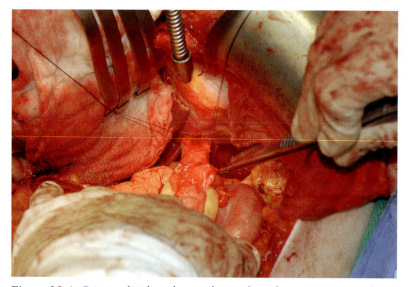

Figure 19-4. Prior to dividing the esophagus, lateral stay sutures are placed to secure the esophagus and prevent retraction into the mediastinum. At least 5-6 cm of esophagus will need to be mobilized below the diaphragmatic hiatus in order to perform a stapled anastamosis safely. The esophagus should be divided sharply and with care to preserve the posterior wall length. A right-angled scalpel blade handle can be useful to perform an esophageal transection that is perpendicular.

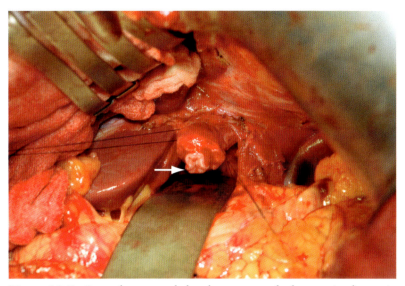

Figure 19-5. Once the stomach has been resected, the proximal margin should be sent for frozen section. No reconstruction should proceed until the surgical team is satisfied with the margin result, as takedown of an esophageal anastamosis wastes esophageal length. Although the esophagus does not have a true serosal layer, there is clearly a mucosal and submucosal layer (arrow), which can separate from the outer muscular layers. Any anastamosis must incorporate all layers of the esophageal wall.

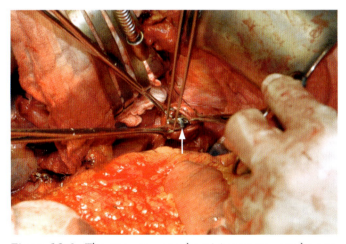

Figure 19-6. The roux-en-y esophagojejunostomy can be performed either by hand-sewn anastamosis or end-end stapled anastamosis (EEA). If EEA is selected, the esophageal lumen is sized and an appropriate stapler is selected. The esophagus may exhibit spasm, and irrigation with warm saline and gentle dilation will help relax the esophagus to accept the EEA anvil (arrow). The anvil is secured with a purse-string suture, which can be hand-sewn or placed with a stapling device. Care should be taken not to tear the esophagus and to perform full-thickness sutures.

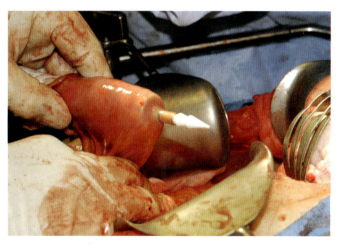

Figure 19-7. The roux limb is placed into position to ensure that the esophagojejunal anastamosis will not be under tension. The stapled end of the roux limb is then resected and the EEA stapler is placed such that the anastamosis will be located on the anti-mesenteric border.

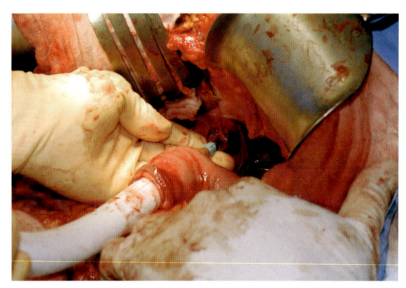

Figure 19-8. The EEA stapler is secured to the esophageal anvil under direct visualization. It is important to orient the roux limb properly so that the anastamosis is not twisted. The EEA stapler is then tightened and fired and carefully removed so as not to put undue tension on the anastamosis. The open end of the roux limb can then be stapled or hand-sewn to complete the roux-en-y gastrojejunostomy.

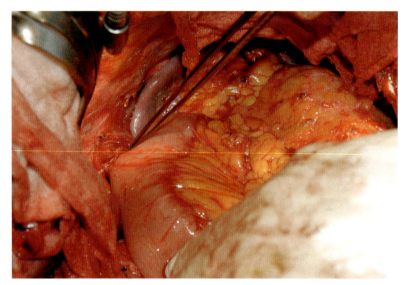

Figure 19-9. After the anastamosis is completed, it can be inspected circumferentially by visual inspection. Suture reinforcement of the anastamosis is acceptable but not necessary, and care should be used to not further constrict the anastamosis. The roux limb should be secured to the diaphragmatic crura to prevent twisting and retraction of the anastamosis into the mediastinum.

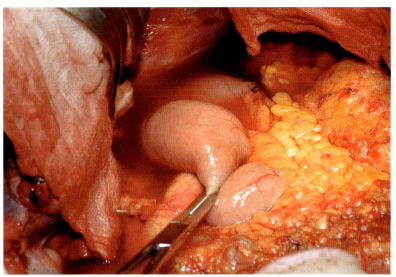

Figure 19-10. A leak test should be performed by gently clamping the roux limb and insufflating air into the distal esophagus either by endoscope or nasogatric tube. Any sign of air leak mandates inspection of the anastamosis with reinforcement of the staple line. A closed suction drain can be placed adjacent to the anastamosis and a feeding jejunostomy can be considered for post-operative enteral nutrition.

Step 5: Pearls and Pitfalls

- It is critically important to accurately stage the tumor preoperatively to determine whether the resection can be done from a strictly abdominal approach.
- En bloc resection of associated organs (distal pancreatectomy, resection of colonic mesentery) can be performed if the tumor directly invades these structures but will result in increased surgical morbidity.
- Pay careful attention to the aspects of the technique regarding esophageal transaction and anastomosis. It is virtually impossible to resect an esophagojejunal anastomosis and perform a second anastomosis all from an abdominal incision.
- If the patient develops a leak of the esophagojejunal anastomosis, the treatment can vary depending upon whether it is detected within the first 48 hours (reexplore, repair leak, and drain), the patient has no evidence of sepsis, and the leak is completely drained externally (continue drainage and jejunal feeds and repeat contrast study in 1 week).

CHAPTER 20

ROUX-EN-Y GASTRIC BYPASS

Leena Khaitan, MD, MPH

Step 1: Surgical Anatomy

- Preoperatively, the patient's upper gastrointestinal anatomy should be evaluated. Screen the patient for symptoms of reflux, dysphagia, or peptic ulcer disease. The patient should undergo an upper endoscopy or barium swallow to evaluate for a hiatal hernia.

Step 2: Preoperative Considerations

- The patient's height and weight should be measured accurately in the office by the surgeon to determine the patient's body mass index (BMI). The patient's BMI should fall within the National Institutes of Health guidelines for weight loss surgery. The BMI should be greater than 40 kg/m^2, or >35 kg/m^2 with an obesity-associated comorbidity.
- All patients should be asked to stop smoking prior to any weight loss procedure. Smoking will impede healing and increase the risk of perioperative pulmonary complications. Furthermore, smoking is currently the number one cause of preventable death. There is no indication to correct the second cause, obesity, if the first one will already result in early mortality.
- Patients should undergo psychologic evaluation to rule out a binge eating disorder. The psychologist or psychiatrist can also help assess the patient's readiness for surgery and determine if the patient has realistic expectations from the surgery. The patient should have a nutritional evaluation and a thorough medical evaluation prior to surgery.
- Review the potential complications with the patient in detail, including the risk of anastomotic leak and death. Every patient's perioperative risk will vary depending on his or her comorbidities.
- The patient should be well educated about the dietary and lifestyle changes that will be required for successful, sustained weight loss. The patient should know and prepare for the modified diet he or she will follow after the surgery.
- It is helpful to advise the patient to lose weight prior to surgery to facilitate the operative procedure. One option is to require patients to lose 10 lbs between their first clinic visit and the surgery date. Placing patients on a liquid diet for 2 weeks prior to the surgery is also advisable. This helps to shrink the visceral fat and particularly the fatty deposits within the liver.

- Have an operating room team that is familiar with bariatric surgery. The nurses should be familiar with the steps of the procedure. The anesthesiologist should be aware of the aggressive fluid resuscitation the patient will require intraoperatively and be skilled at difficult intubations.
- Patients receive a bowel prep the day prior to the procedure.
- On the day of the procedure patients receive prophylactic antibiotics. Patients receive deep venous thrombosis prophylaxis with sequential compression devices and subcutaneous or fractionated heparin.

Step 3: Operative Steps

1. **Room Setup** (Figure 20-1)

- The patient is positioned supine on the bed. The feet are secured to a footboard and both arms are left out. Care should be taken to be sure the arms are well padded to avoid a brachial plexus injury. The feet should be positioned flat on the footboard and secured so that they cannot supinate or pronate. A Foley catheter should be placed prior to positioning. The surgeon stands to the right side of the patient. The assistant stands to the left of the patient and will also operate the camera.

2. **Port Placement** (Figure 20-1)

- The patient's prior surgical history should be assessed prior to port placement. If the patient has no prior history of surgery in the left upper quadrant, then this area is used as the point of initial entry. An optical trocar is used to enter the peritoneal cavity under direct visualization. Due to the thickness of the abdominal wall, a direct Hasson approach may be challenging.
- The camera port is measured 21 cm from the xiphoid process and positioned just to the left of midline. An imaginary line is drawn from this point to the junction of the left costal margin and midclavicular line. The initial port, a 12-mm bladeless optical trocar that allows direct visualization as one enters the peritoneal cavity, is placed at the midpoint of this line in the left upper quadrant.. This port will serve as the surgeon's right hand. The abdomen is insufflated to 15 mm Hg, and a 30-degree scope is inserted through this port.
- Three additional trocars are placed. A 10-mm trocar is placed at the previously determined site near the midline (for the camera). A 12-mm trocar is placed four fingerbreadths from the xiphoid process off of the right costal margin and is directed to the patient's left, so that it enters the peritoneal cavity off the tip of the left lobe of the liver and falciform ligament junction (for the surgeon's left hand). A 5-mm trocar is placed in the left anterior axillary line just below the left costal margin (for the assistant).

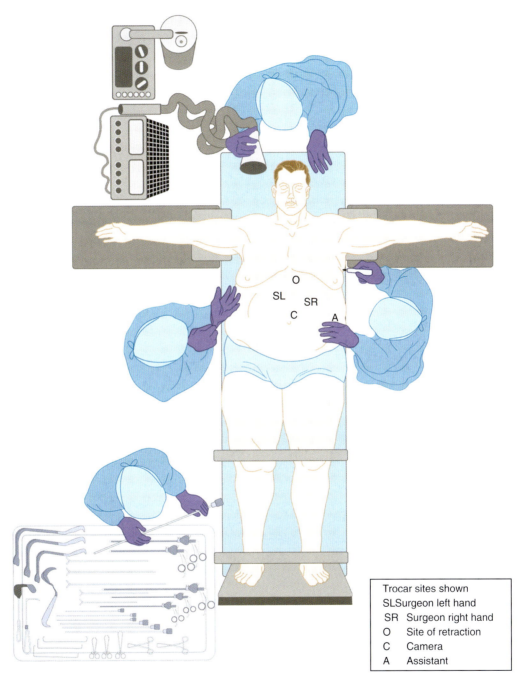

Trocar sites shown
SL Surgeon left hand
SR Surgeon right hand
O   Site of retraction
C   Camera
A   Assistant

Figure 20-1

3. Dissection into Lesser Sac (Figure 20-2)

- The lesser sac is entered along the body of the greater curvature of the stomach using a harmonic scalpel to avoid bleeding from the short gastrics. The opening is made about 2 to 3 cm in diameter.

4. Creation of Jejunojejunostomy

- The omentum is lifted up and over the transverse colon and placed in the upper abdomen, exposing the ligament of Treitz. The small bowel is rotated from this point in a clockwise fashion for a distance of 30 cm, and this site is chosen to divide the jejunum. Using blunt dissection, a DeBakey-tipped grasper is used to dissect through the mesentery in the avascular plane next to the bowel. A blue cartridge stapler is then passed through the dissected area and around the bowel, and the bowel is divided. (Figure 20-3) The harmonic scalpel is then used to divide the mesentery toward its base. (Figure 20-4) A small Penrose drain is sutured to the distal cut end of bowel with a 2-0 silk suture to mark it for later in the procedure. (Figure 20-5)
- The distal bowel (future Roux limb) is then rotated in a counterclockwise fashion for a distance of 150 cm, and this site is chosen for the jejunojejunostomy. The biliopancreatic limb and this distal end of the Roux limb are sutured together using a 2-0 silk suture placed at the distal end of the future anastomosis.

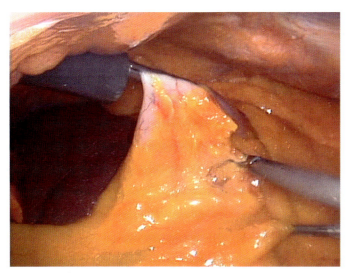

Figure 20-2

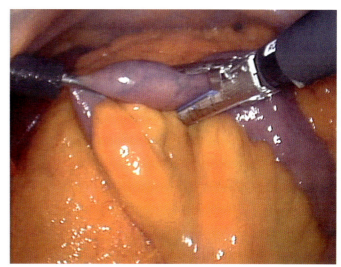

Figure 20-3

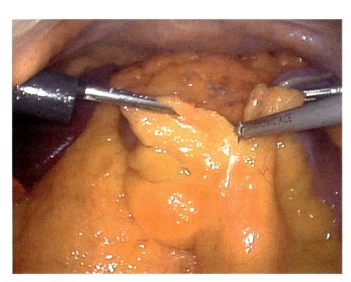

Figure 20-4

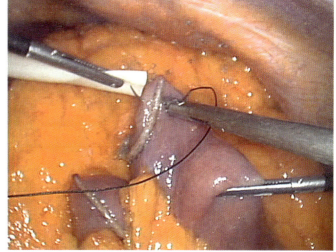

Figure 20-5

- The assistant holds this suture, and the surgeon creates an enterotomy in each limb of bowel using the harmonic scalpel. Care is taken to make these enterotomies only large enough to accommodate the stapler. (Figure 20-6) A white cartridge stapler is then passed through the right upper quadrant port and roticulated anteriorly. (Figure 20-7) A side-to-side, functional end-to-end anastomosis is created.
- The common enterotomy is then held closed using three stay sutures. (Figure 20-8) Two are held by the assistant and one is held by the surgeon. The enterotomy is then stapled closed using a blue cartridge stapler. The staple line is then inspected carefully to ensure a good closure.
- The mesenteric defect is closed carefully using a running suture with a Lapra-Ty (Ethicon, Cincinnati, OH) at either end to prevent future internal hernias. (Figure 20-9)

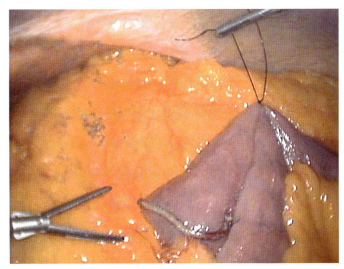

Figure 20-6

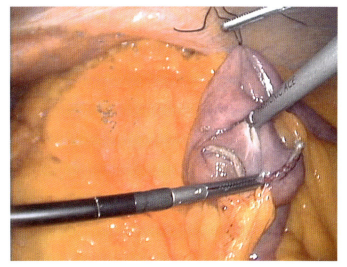

Figure 20-7

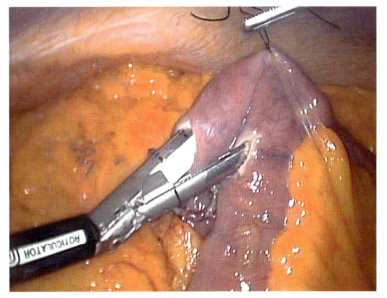

Figure 20-8

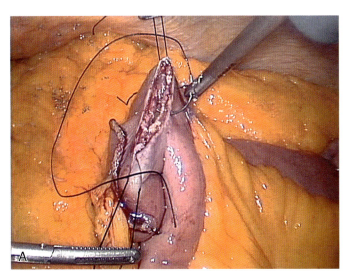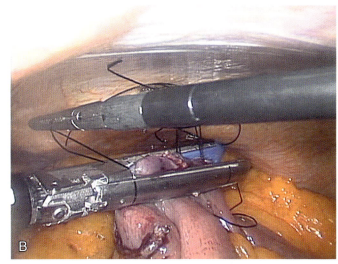

Figure 20-9

5. Passage of the Roux Limb

- Attention is turned to the transverse colon mesentery, and the "bare" area is identified lateral to the middle colic vessels. It is incised using the harmonic scalpel to enter the lesser sac. The proximal end of the Roux limb is passed retrocolic into the lesser sac. (Figure 20-10) The entry into the lesser sac along the greater curvature of the stomach is used to then bring the proximal Roux limb into the antigastric position. The proximal end should face the left side of the patient and come up easily without any tension so that the mesentery is not twisted. (Figure 20-11)

6. Creation of the Pouch

- The patient is placed in the steep reverse Trendelenburg position, and the Nathanson retractor is placed just to the left of the xiphoid process in the mid epigastrium. This is a curved retractor that is manipulated beneath the left lobe of the liver to expose the esophageal hiatus and is held in place by a self-retaining retractor affixed to the side of the bed. (Figure 20-12)
- Dissection is begun on the lesser curve five centimeters from the GE junction. This will be the inferior aspect of the gastric pouch. Blunt and ultrasonic dissection is used to enter the lesser sac. Care is taken to preserve the vagal nerves. (Figure 20-13)
- A gastrotomy is made on the body of the stomach distal to the future pouch. The left upper quadrant incision is extended, and the anvil for a 25-mm EEA stapler (Ethicon) is passed into the peritoneal cavity. A wound protector is then placed at this trocar site, and the trocar replaced.

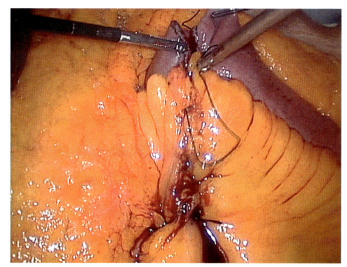

Figure 20-10

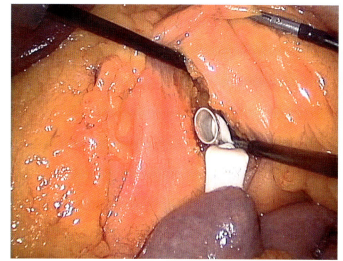

Figure 20-11

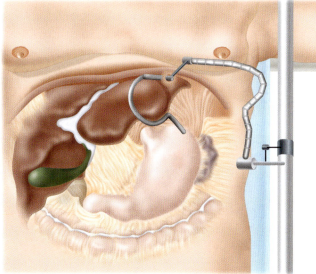

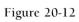

Figure 20-12

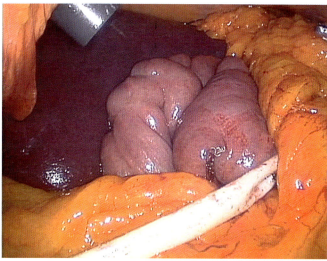

Figure 20-13

- An anvil grasper is used to pass the anvil through the gastrotomy to the site of the future gastrojejunostomy. This should be just above the entry point into the lesser sac on the lesser curvature of the stomach (Figure 20-14) The gastrotomy is then closed using the blue or green cartridge stapler, depending on the thickness of the stomach.
- The pouch is then created around the anvil. A single transverse staple line is placed just below the anvil where the entry into the lesser sac was made. Then the pouch is completed by stapling up toward the angle of His. A reinforcement along the staple line (Seamguard, Gore) can be helpful in minimizing staple-line bleeding and has been shown to decrease leaks in some studies. An Ewald tube is passed into the pouch prior to each vertical staple firing to help size the pouch and to avoid stapling across the gastroesophageal junction. (Figure 20-15) Care should be taken to ensure that the pouch and remnant are completely divided.

7. Creation of the Gastrojejunostomy

- Attention is turned to the proximal end of the Roux limb. An enterotomy is made at the staple line large enough to allow passage of a 25-mm EEA. The spike is removed from the anvil, and the EEA is passed through the left upper quadrant incision into the peritoneal cavity and into the enterotomy for a distance of 3 to 4 cm. This is facilitated by the assistant who has firmly grasped the proximal end of the roux limb. (Figure 20-16) The spike is brought through the antimesenteric side of the jejunum. Both the 25-mm EEA and anvil are mated, creating a circular stapled anastomosis. An anvil grasper is useful to have since the anvil is difficult to grasp with most atraumatic graspers. The EEA is removed and the donuts are checked for completeness. (Figure 20-17)
- The mesentery is divided on the excess jejunum and the enterotomy is stapled closed. The excess bowel is removed. (Figure 20-18) The anastomosis is oversewn with Medtronic U-clips. (Figure 20-19)
- An intraoperative leak test is performed by insufflating the pouch endoscopically and filling the peritoneal cavity with saline. If any air bubbles are seen, the staple line is oversewn until there are no leaks. This is a rare event but very important to recognize.

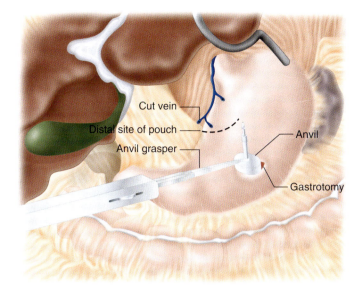

Figure 20-14

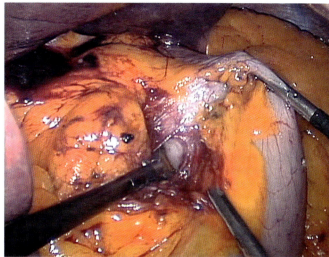

Figure 20-15

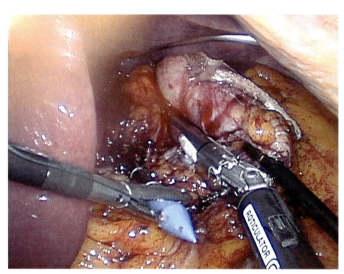

Figure 20-16

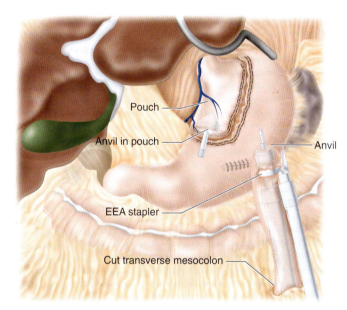

Figure 20-17

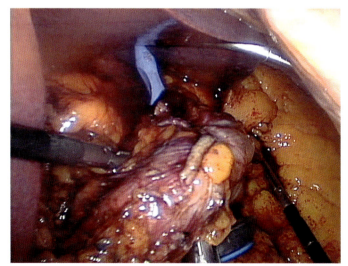

Figure 20-18

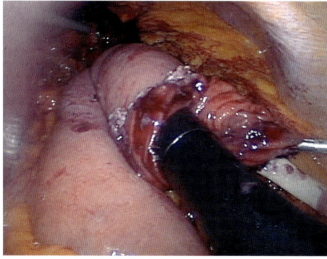

Figure 20-19

8. **Closure**

- The transverse mesocolon defect is closed with a continuous permanent suture. To save time, a Lapra-Ty is used to secure the suture in place at either end.
- Final anatomy undergoes a final visual inspection. (Figure 20-20)
- A drain is placed through the 5-mm trocar site and placed in the left upper quadrant next to the staple line.
- The left upper quadrant incision is closed using 0-Vicryl sutures placed in figure-of-8 fashion using the laparoscopic suture passer.
- The abdomen is deflated, and the other trocars are removed. The incisions are closed using a running subcuticular suture with 4-0 polyglactin 910.
- Dermabond is placed on the wounds.

Step 4: Postoperative Care

- Patients should be aggressively hydrated throughout the procedure and postoperatively to maintain at least 0.5 cc/kg/hour. For the morbidly obese patient, this can be 75 cc or more.
- Early ambulation on the day of surgery is paramount along with DVT prophylaxis in preventing complications of thromboembolism. Ambulation along with incentive spirometry helps to minimize atelectasis and postoperative pulmonary complications.
- Diabetics should be placed on a sliding scale as their insulin requirements are likely to drop following surgery.
- On postoperative day 1, a gastrograffin swallow is obtained to further confirm the absence of a leak at the gastrojejunostomy.
- On postoperative day 1, if the patient is clinically doing well and the swallow is negative, then the liquid diet can be started. The patient starts on 1 oz of water or juice every hour for 4 hours and then increases up to 4 oz/hour thereafter. On postoperative day 2, the patient increases oral intake by 1 oz/hour up to 8 oz/hour. At this point the patient can resume necessary meds orally with the medication crushed or in a liquid form.
- The patient is discharged to home on postoperative day 2 on a liquid diet. Patients will remain on liquids for 1 week, then progress to pureed food. At 1 month the patient can increase consistency to soft foods.

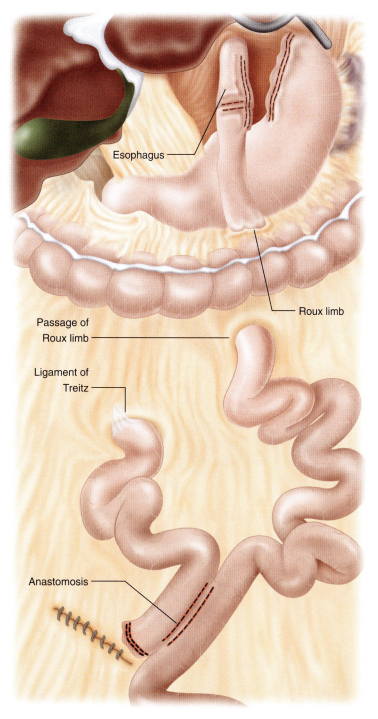

Esophagus

Roux limb

Passage of
Roux limb

Ligament of
Treitz

Anastomosis

Figure 20-20

Step 5: Pearls and Pitfalls

- As with any surgical procedure, patient selection is the key to a good outcome. Patients should be thoroughly evaluated preoperatively for sleep apnea with a sleep study, cardiac problems with EKG and Stress Echo, pulmonary function tests, and psychologic evaluation. Early in one's experience, patients over the age of 60 and BMI >55 kg/m^2 should be avoided as they are known to be associated with a higher morbidity rate.
- Close communication with the anesthesiologist and aggressive intraoperative resuscitation can set the stage for an uneventful recovery. The patients have undergone a bowel prep prior to surgery and come to the operating room dehydrated. Usually a goal of around 4 L of intravenous fluids intraoperatively will help to avoid multiple bolus requirements in the postoperative period.
- Careful monitoring of patient heart rate and urine output can alert the surgeon early of a postoperative complication. Many studies have shown that sustained tachycardia (heart rate > 100 bpm for over 3 to 4 hours) is the best predictor of a postoperative anastomotic leak. If for any reason the patient's recovery deviates from the expected clinical course, a high index of suspicion and aggressive return to the operating room for reexploration is mandated. This will facilitate early intervention if the patient does have an anastomotic leak that was not recognized at the time of surgery and avoid even worse consequences.
- Extensive nutritional and exercise counseling preoperatively is very helpful in the patient's postoperative care. Many lifestyle changes such as avoiding sodas, taking vitamins, and incorporating daily exercise time into the patient's routine can be done prior to surgery. This will make it easier for the patient to adopt the other required lifestyle changes postoperatively.
- When making the enterotomies in the jejunal limbs for the jejunojejunostomy, do not make them too big. Otherwise, closure of the enterotomy may lead to a stricture in this area. If the enterotomy is large, then the anastomosis should be created with two firings of the stapler (90-mm staple line) to prevent stricture.

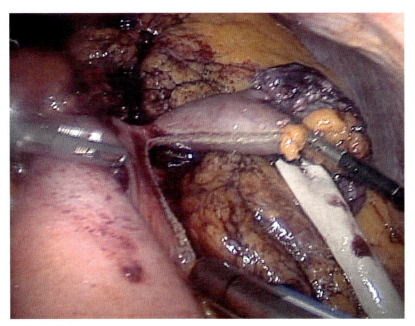

Figure 20-21

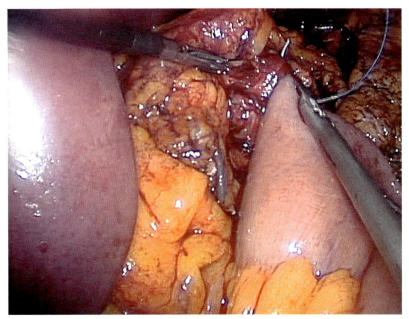

Figure 20-22

- When creating the gastric pouch around the anvil, it is helpful to have the anesthesiologist move the Ewald tube into and out of the pouch before firing the stapler.
- Although a drain is not necessary at the end of the procedure, it is helpful in draining fluid from the leak test and also potentially controlling a leak if one occurs. It is usually removed prior to the patient's discharge from the hospital.
- If the patient is on several medications, consider placing a gastrostomy tube in the remnant stomach that can be removed when the patient comes off of some of their medications and can tolerate the rest of them by mouth. Many medications are unpalatable when crushed and may be difficult for the patient to tolerate initially following surgery.

References

1. Colquitt J, Clegg A, Loveman E, et al. Surgery for morbid obesity. *Cochrane Database Syst Rev* 2005; Oct 19;(4):CD003641.
2. Farrell TM, Haggerty SP, Overby DW, et al. Clinical application of laparoscopic bariatric surgery: an evidence-based review. *Surg Endosc* 2009; 23(5):930-949.
3. Puzziferri N, Austrheim-Smith IT, Wolfe BM, et al. Three-year follow-up of a prospective randomized trial comparing laparoscopic versus open gastric bypass. *Ann Surg* 2006; 243(2):181-188.

CHAPTER 21

GASTRIC BAND

Leena Khaitan, MD, MPH

Step 1: Surgical Anatomy

- The gastric band is placed at the upper portion of the stomach just distal to the gastroesophageal junction, at around the level of the first or second vein on the lesser curve of the stomach.
- In order to access this area of the abdomen, the left lobe of the liver must be retracted anteriorly throughout the procedure.
- The base of the crura can be identified by opening the clear area of the gastrohepatic omentum and retracting the lesser curve of the stomach laterally.
- The angle of His can be identified along the left crus. The omental fat at the fundus of the stomach is retracted caudally, and the fundus is retracted medially to identify the angle and the left crus.

Step 2: Preoperative Considerations

- The patient's height and weight should be measured accurately in the office by the surgeon to determine the patient's body mass index (BMI). The patient's BMI should fall within the NIH guidelines for weight loss surgery. The BMI should be greater than 40 kg/m^2 or ≤35 kg/m^2 with a comorbidity.
- Patients should undergo psychologic evaluation to rule out a binge eating disorder. The psychologist/psychiatrist can also help assess the patient's readiness for surgery and determine if the patient has realistic expectations from the surgery. The patient should have a nutritional evaluation and a thorough medical evaluation prior to surgery.
- All patients should be asked to stop smoking prior to any weight loss procedure. Smoking will impede healing and increase the risk of perioperative pulmonary complications. Furthermore, smoking is currently the number one cause of preventable death. There is no indication to correct the second cause, obesity, if the first one will already result in early mortality.
- The patient should be well educated about the dietary and lifestyle changes that will be required for successful, sustained weight loss. The patient should know and prepare for the modified diet he or she will follow after the surgery. Patients are counseled on how to incorporate exercise into his or her daily schedules to achieve 1 hour of exercise 5 to 7 days per week.

- It is helpful to advise the patient to lose weight prior to surgery to help facilitate the operative procedure. One option is to require patients to lose 10 lbs and to place them on a liquid diet for 2 weeks prior to the surgery. This helps to shrink the visceral fat and particularly the fatty deposits within the liver.
- The patient should be evaluated for the presence of a hiatal hernia preoperatively to adequately prepare for the procedure. If a moderate to large hiatal hernia (>2 cm) is present, consider repairing it at the time of placement of the band.

Step 3: Operative Steps

1. Room Setup (Figure 21-1)

- The patient is positioned supine on the bed. The feet are secured to a footboard, and both arms are left out. Care should be taken to be sure the arms are well padded to avoid a brachial plexus injury. The feet should be positioned flat on the footboard and secured so that they cannot supinate or pronate.
- The surgeon stands to the right side of the patient. The assistant stands to the left of the patient and will also operate the camera.

2. Port Placement (Figure 21-1)

- The patient's prior surgical history should be assessed prior to port placement. If the patient has no prior history of surgery in the left upper quadrant, then this area is used as the point of initial entry. An optical trocar is used to enter the peritoneal cavity under direct visualization. Due to the thickness of the abdominal wall, a direct Hasson approach with a cut-down may be challenging.
- Measurement is made 12 cm from the xiphoid process in the midline and the point lateral to this, and just medial to the midclavicular line in the left upper quadrant is used for the initial 10-mm port. A #11 blade is used to make a 1-cm incision, and the trocar is inserted. The abdomen is then insufflated with CO_2 to 15 mm Hg.
- Three additional trocars are placed. A 15-mm bladeless trocar is placed under direct visualization just to the right of midline lateral to the previously marked point 12 cm below the xiphoid. This trocar is placed at an angle so that it comes through the base of the falciform ligament.
- The remaining two trocars are 5 mm. One is placed in the anterior axillary line just below the left costal margin for the assistant. The other is placed in the right upper quadrant off of the tip of the right lobe of the liver for the surgeon's left hand. This port may need to be placed slightly more medially depending on the size of the patient. This positioning of the trocar will be in direct line of the dissection plane posterior to the stomach. The graspers should be able to reach the left upper quadrant comfortably. Both are placed under direct visualization after anesthetizing the area with 0.5% bupivacaine (Marcaine). (Figure 21-1)

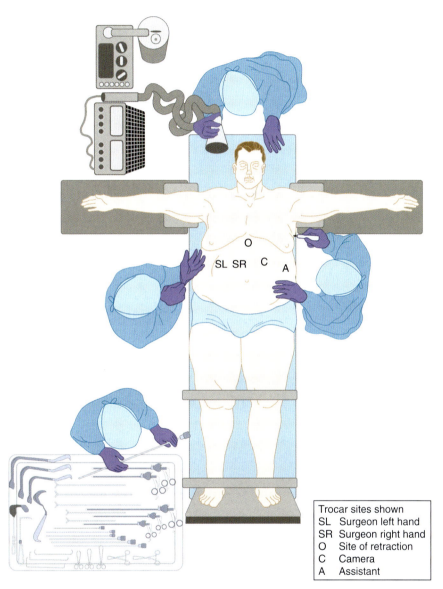

Trocar sites shown
SL Surgeon left hand
SR Surgeon right hand
O   Site of retraction
C   Camera
A   Assistant

Figure 21-1

◆ Finally a Nathanson retractor is placed to elevate the left lobe of the liver and expose the gas-troesophageal junction. A small incision is made just to the left of xiphoid, and the obturator for a 5-mm trocar is placed perpendicular to the skin toward the level of the peritoneum but not through the peritoneum. Then, through the same tract, the Nathanson retractor is passed and manipulated into place below the left lobe of the liver. This retractor is held in place using a self-retaining mechanical arm affixed to the left side of the patient's bed. (Figure 21-2)

3. Dissection

◆ Dissection is begun at the angle of His (Figure 21-3). The assistant places his or her grasper over the omental fat of the fundus and sweeps it caudally toward the feet. A Ray-tec may be helpful for this maneuver. Care is taken to avoid too much traction on the spleen. The surgeon the retracts the fundus further caudad using the grasper through the furthest right port to expose the angle of His. Blunt and cautery dissection using the hook dissector is used to dissect along the gastroesophageal junction to the base of the left crus.

◆ If the patient has a very prominent phrenoesophageal fat pad, this should be dissected off of the stomach in a cephalad fashion using blunt, ultrasonic, and/or cautery dissection, depending on the surgeon's choice. The fat pad can be completely excised for even better exposure in patients with larger BMI's. This will allow the portion of the stomach encircled by the band to be less likely to be obstructed by the placement of the band.

◆ Then attention is turned to the lesser curve of the stomach. The clear portion of the gastrohe-patic omentum (pars flaccida) is incised. (Figure 21-4) The stomach is retracted laterally by the assistant to expose the right crus down toward the base of the crural junction. (Figure 21-5) Very limited cautery is applied at this site and then the grasper in the surgeon's left hand is passed through this area into the left upper quadrant to the already dissected angle of His. The grasper should pass very smoothly without resistance. (Figure 21-6)

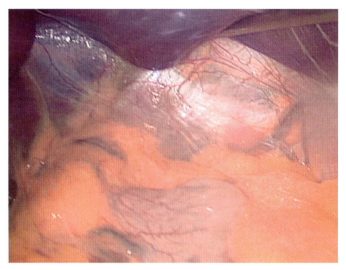

Figure 21-2

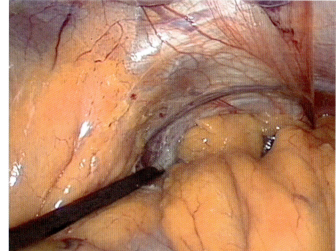

Figure 21-3

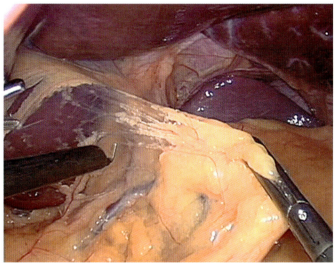

Figure 21-4

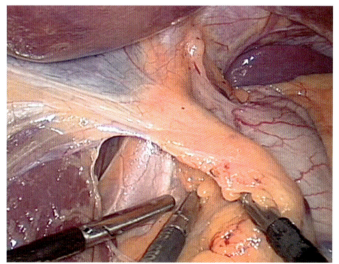

Figure 21-5

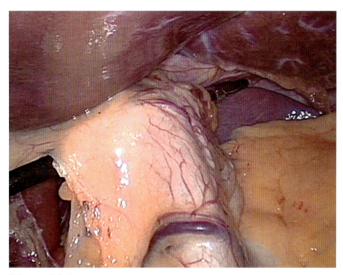

Figure 21-6

4. Placement of Band into the Abdomen

- The band is flushed with saline prior to placement into the peritoneal cavity. The end of the band itself is grasped with the DeBakey grasper and passed through the 15-mm trocar into the peritoneal cavity. The grasper is removed, and the end of the tubing is passed through this same trocar into the abdomen so that the entire band is in the abdomen. (Figure 21-2)
- The end of the tubing is then handed to the grasper, which is still sitting in the left upper quadrant (Figure 21-7) and pulled around the back of the stomach. When the band itself is coming around, do not pull so hard that the entire band comes through. The most difficult portion of the band to bring through is the shoulders. (Figure 21-8)
- Pass the tubing through the buckle on the band and buckle the band in place. (Figure 21-9) The band can now be sewn in place. The assistant should retract the tubing of the band toward the 7 o'clock position to provide optimal visualization for the surgeon.
- Simple sutures are placed to plicate the fundus over the anterior portion of the band to hold it in place. This plication begins on the greater curve as far laterally as possible and progresses toward the lesser curve. (Figure 21-10) Typically three to four sutures are placed with careful apposition of gastric serosa to gastric serosa. This should not be sewn to the esophagus. The sutures should stop before any stomach is placed over the buckle of the band to minimize risk of erosion. (Figure 21-11)

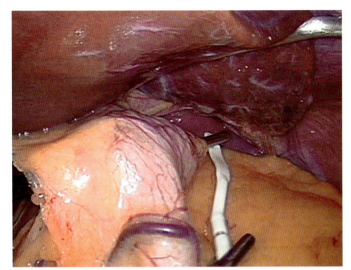

Figure 21-7

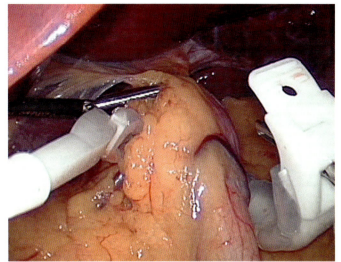

Figure 21-8

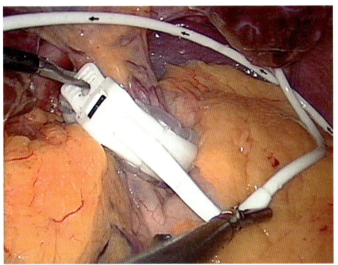

Figure 21-9

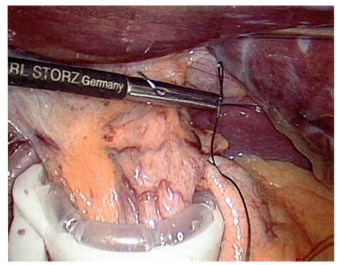

Figure 21-10

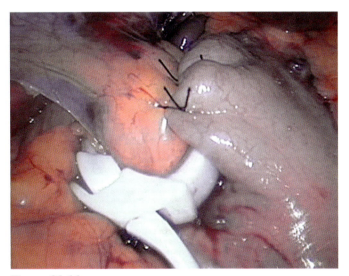

Figure 21-11

5. Securing Port (Figure 21-12)

- The end of the tubing is grasped and brought through the 15-mm port to the outside of the abdominal wall. The Nathanson retractor and the other trocars are removed under direct visualization, and the abdomen is deflated.
- The port is attached to the externalized tubing, and then a pocket is dissected in the subcutaneous tissues cephalad and medial to the 15-mm incision, so that the port can sit in the mid epigastrium. This is the thinnest part of the abdominal wall, which will facilitate future adjustments.
- Four 0-prolene or other nonabsorbable sutures are placed at the corners of a square and then placed through the fixation holes of the port. Access to the anterior fascia can be difficult and long narrow retractors are needed. Schofield retractors are very helpful. If you do not have these then long, narrow Deaver retractors or appendiceal retractors can be used. The port is parachuted down to the anterior fascia and secured in place. The port should be placed far enough from the 15-mm trocar site such that it lays flat on the fascia. The excess tubing is directed back into the abdominal cavity. The tubing should be left long so that it does not act like an adhesive band within the peritoneal cavity.

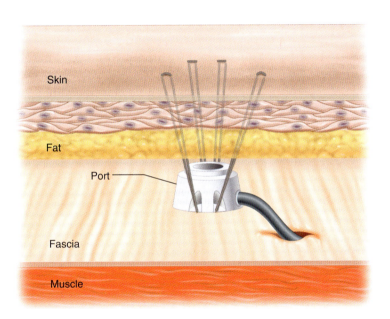

Figure 21-12

6. Closure

- All ports are closed at the level of the skin with 4-0 absorbable sutures placed in a subcuticular fashion. No fascial closure is performed at any of the port sites. The 15-mm port site is closed in two layers. Interrupted 3-0 polyglactin 910 sutures are used to close the Scarpa fascia, and then skin is closed. A liquid skin adhesive is placed on all of the wounds.

Step 4: Postoperative Care

- Patients are kept overnight for a 23-hour stay and to ensure that they can tolerate enough oral intake to avoid dehydration when discharged. They are NPO on the day of surgery and then are started on a liquid diet on postoperative day 1. The patient is started on 1 oz of clear liquids/hour and then slowly progressed to 4 oz/hour.
- Patients are visited by the nutritionist prior to discharge to review and reinforce the postoperative diet.
- Patients are maintained on DVT prophylaxis with sequential compression device's and subcutaneous heparin. Patients are ambulated on the day of surgery to minimize venous thromboembolism risk.
- Patients should be aggressively hydrated during and after the procedure to maintain at least 0.5 cc/kg/hour urine output. The patient's fluid status needs to be closely monitored.
- All medications are crushed or in a liquid form for at least the first month following surgery.
- No adjustments of the band are done for at least 6 weeks following the procedure.

Step 5: Pearls and Pitfalls

- Patients should be very well educated regarding the new tool they have been given. The greatest benefit of the band is that the patients are no longer hungry. The band will not give them dumping and therefore will not prevent the patient from consuming unneeded liquid calories. Once the patients are able to be advanced to a solid diet, recommend that the majority of the protein nutrition they take in should be in a solid form. This is what will keep them feeling full.
- When dissecting posterior to the stomach to pass the grasper, there should be minimal bleeding and minimal resistance. If either of these situations occur, the surgeon should reevaluate their plane of dissection.
- Take care to be sure the port is secured firmly to the fascia. Very good retractors will facilitate this portion of the procedure. Schofield retractors are better than Deavers or appendiceal retractors. This is often the most time-consuming and challenging portion of the operation. The sutures should be placed in four corners and then threaded through the sites on the port. The port should be parachuted down to the fascia and fixed in place.
- The real work for the surgeon with this procedure is not the procedure itself but the before and after care of the patient. It is important to be familiar with the different band adjustment strategies to be able to use the one that will work best for patients. Having a nutritionist readily available can also help tremendously in the aftercare of these patients.

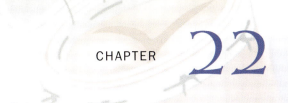
GASTRIC SLEEVE

Leena Khaitan, MD, MPH

Step 1: Surgical Anatomy

- Preoperatively, the patient's upper gastrointestinal anatomy should be evaluated. Screen the patient for symptoms of reflux, dysphagia, or peptic ulcer disease. The patient should undergo an upper endoscopy or barium swallow to evaluate for a hiatal hernia.

Step 2: Preoperative Considerations

- This procedure is currently mostly reserved for those patients who are super obese or who may be high risk for a gastric bypass procedure. The sleeve gastrectomy can be used as a staging procedure for a future gastric bypass or duodenal switch. It works as a restrictive-only procedure.
- The patient's height and weight should be measured accurately in the office by the surgeon to determine the patient's body mass index (BMI). The patient's BMI should fall within the NIH guidelines for weight loss surgery. The BMI should be greater than 40 kg/m² or >35 kg/m² with an obesity-associated comorbidity.
- All patients should be asked to stop smoking prior to any weight loss procedure. Smoking will impede healing and increase risk of perioperative pulmonary complications. Furthermore, smoking is currently the number one cause of preventable death. There is no indication to correct the second cause, obesity, if the first one will already result in early mortality.
- Patients should undergo psychologic evaluation to rule out a binge eating disorder. The psychologist or psychiatrist can also help assess the patient's readiness for surgery and determine if the patient has realistic expectations from the surgery. The patient should have a nutritional evaluation and a thorough medical evaluation prior to surgery.
- Review the potential complications with the patient in detail including risk of anastomotic leak and death. Every patient's perioperative risk will vary depending on his or her comorbidities.
- The patient should be well educated about the dietary and lifestyle changes that will be required for successful, sustained weight loss. The patient should know and prepare for the modified diet he or she will follow after the surgery.
- It is helpful to advise the patient to lose weight prior to surgery to help facilitate the operative procedure. One option is to require patients to lose 10 lbs between their first clinic visit and the surgery date. Placing patients on a liquid diet for 2 weeks prior to the surgery is also advisable. This helps to shrink the visceral fat and particularly the fatty deposits within the liver.

- Have an operating room team that is familiar with bariatric surgery. The nurses should be familiar with the steps of the procedure. The anesthesiologist should be aware of the aggressive fluid resuscitation the patient will require intraoperatively and be skilled at difficult intubations.
- Patients receive a bowel prep the day prior to the procedure.
- On the day of the procedure patients receive prophylactic antibiotics. Patients receive deep venous thrombosis prophylaxis with sequential compression devices and subcutaneous or fractionated heparin.

Step 3: Operative Steps

1. Room Setup (Figure 22-1)

- The patient is positioned supine on the bed. The feet are secured to a footboard, and both arms are left out. Care should be taken to be sure the arms are well padded to avoid a brachial plexus injury. The feet should be positioned flat on the footboard and secured so that they cannot supinate or pronate. A Foley catheter should be placed prior to positioning. The surgeon stands to the right side of the patient. The assistant stands to the left of the patient and will also operate the camera.

2. Port Placement (Figure 22-1)

- The patient's prior surgical history should be assessed prior to port placement. If the patient has no prior history of surgery in the left upper quadrant, then this area is used as the point of initial entry. An optical trocar is used to enter the peritoneal cavity under direct visualization. Due to the thickness of the abdominal wall, a direct Hasson approach may be challenging.
- The ports are placed similar to that of a gastric bypass. The initial 12-mm port is placed in the left upper quadrant medial to the midclavicular line around the level of the base of the rib cage. An optical trocar can be used to access the peritoneal cavity. This port will be the surgeon's right hand and the site through which the stomach remnant will be removed.
- A second 12-mm port is placed four fingerbreadths from the xiphoid process off of the right costal margin.
- The assistant places a 5-mm port in the anterior axillary line off of the left costal margin.
- The camera port is placed 20 cm from the xiphoid just to the left of midline.
- The patient is placed in the steep reverse Trendelenburg position, and the Nathanson retractor is placed just to the left of the xiphoid in the mid epigastrium. This is a curved retractor that is manipulated beneath the left lobe of the liver to expose the esophageal hiatus and is held in place by a self-retaining retractor affixed to the side of the bed.

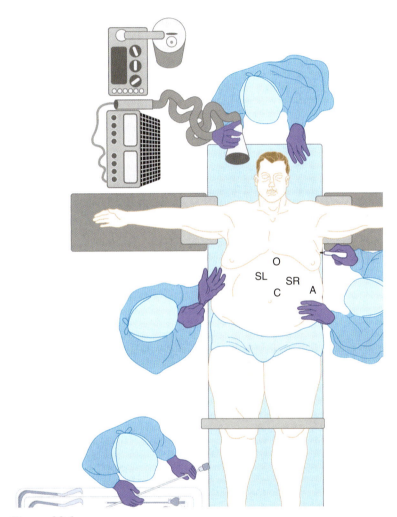

Figure 22-1

3. Procedure

- The procedure is begun by dividing the omentum off of the greater curvature of the stomach, starting at 5 to 6 cm proximal to the pylorus and progressing to the junction of the left crus and angle of His. This can be done using ultrasonic energy or another vessel-sealing device such as LigaSure device (Valley Labs). (Figure 22-2) Meticulous hemostasis should be maintained.
- Next either an endoscope or a 32 Fr bougie is passed into the stomach along the lesser curvature toward the pylorus.
- Sequential firings of a linear stapler along the sizing device will create the future tabularized stomach. The staplers are fired alongside the bougie to ensure a consistently tabularized stomach up toward the gastroesophageal junction and the angle of His. The 3.5-mm or 4.8-mm staplers should be used based on the thickness of the stomach. These staple lines can be reinforced with products such as Seamguard (Gore), or the entire staple line should be oversewn. (Figure 22-3) This will create a 60 to 80 cc gastric tube. The divided stomach is removed through the left upper quadrant incision.
- An intraoperative leak test is performed by insufflating air in the stomach and filling the upper abdomen with saline. Any leaks should be oversewn.

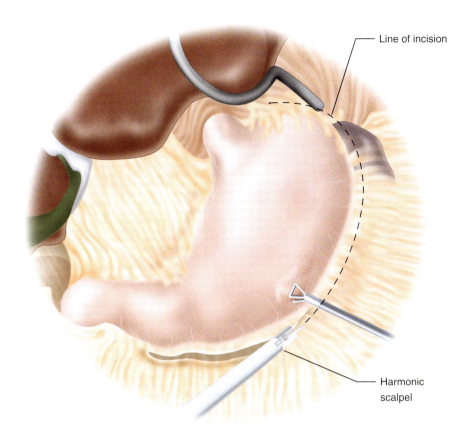

Line of incision

Harmonic
scalpel

Figure 22-2

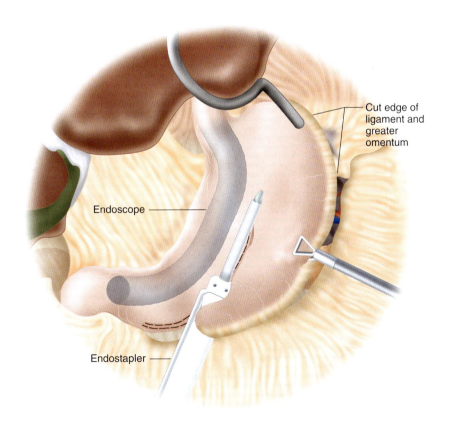

Cut edge of
ligament and
greater
omentum

Endoscope

Endostapler

Figure 22-3

♦ All ports over 10 mm are closed at the level of the fascia using the laparoscopic suture passer in a simple fashion. Skin is closed with 4-0 polyglactin 910 placed in a subcuticular fashion. Dermabond is placed on all of the wounds. (Figure 22-4)

Step 4: Postoperative Care

♦ Patients should be aggressively hydrated throughout the procedure and postoperatively to maintain at least 0.5 cc/kg/hour. For the morbidly obese patient, this can be 75 cc or more.
♦ Early ambulation on the day of surgery is paramount along with DVT prophylaxis in preventing complications of thromboembolism. Ambulation along with incentive spirometry helps to minimize atelectasis and postoperative pulmonary complications.
♦ Diabetics should be placed on a sliding scale as their insulin requirements are likely to drop following surgery.
♦ On postoperative day 1 a gastrograffin swallow is obtained to further confirm the absence of a leak along the staple line.
♦ On postoperative day 1, if the patient is clinically doing well and the swallow is negative, then the liquid diet can be started. The patient starts on 1 oz of water or juice every hour for 4 hours and then increases up to 4 oz/hour thereafter. On postoperative day 2, the patient increases oral intake by 1 oz/hour up to 8 oz/hour. At this point the patient can resume necessary meds orally with the medication crushed or in a liquid form.
♦ The patient is discharged to home on postoperative day 2 on a liquid diet. Patients will remain on liquids for 1 week, then progress to pureed food. At 1 month the patient can increase consistency to soft foods.

Step 5: Pearls and Pitfalls

♦ The vertical gastrectomy should be offered as part of a staging procedure to the patient. This is a restrictive procedure and is reserved for the high-risk patient or patient with BMI >60 kg/m^2.
♦ It can be considered as a primary procedure for patients with lower BMI, although this is still considered investigational.
♦ This can be a reasonable procedure to consider in the elderly. It has a short operative time and relatively few complications compared to the gastric bypass procedure.
♦ This can be used as a staging procedure to the duodenal switch or the gastric bypass in the super obese, leaving options for the surgeon. The average interval to the second stage is around 1 year.

References

1. Farrell TM, Haggerty SP, Overby DW, et al. Clinical application of laparoscopic bariatric surgery: an evidence-based review. *Surg Endosc* 2009; 23(5):1125-1129.
2. Karamanakos SN, Vagenas K, Kalfarentzos F, et al. Weight loss, appetite suppression, and changes in fasting and postprandial ghrelin and peptide-YY levels after Roux-en-Y gastric bypass and sleeve gastrectomy: a prospective, double blind study. *Ann Surg* 2008; 247(3):401-407.
3. Moy J, Pomp A, Dakin G, et al. Laparoscopic sleeve gastrectomy for morbid obesity. *Am J Surg* 2008; 196(5):e56-e59.
4. Tucker ON, Szomstein S, Rosenthal RJ. Indications for sleeve gastrectomy as a primary procedure for weight loss in the morbidly obese. *J Gastrointest Surg* 2008; 12(4):662-667.

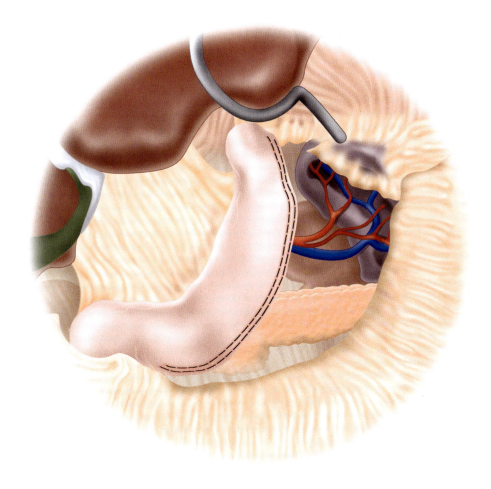

Figure 22-4

CHAPTER 23

SMALL BOWEL RESECTION AND ANASTOMOSIS

Bradley Champagne, MD

Step 1: Surgical Anatomy

- The submucosal layer of the bowel is the strongest layer of the intestines, and regardless of the anastomotic technique must be incorporated in all anastomosis.

Step 2: Preoperative Considerations

- The technique for small bowel resection varies depending on the clinical presentation, intraoperative findings, and location along the alimentary tract. It is preferable to utilize both stapled and hand-sewn techniques. Stapled anastomosis can be performed rapidly, accurately, and with a lower leak rate than hand-sewn anastomosis in some series. However, when there is a discrepancy in diameter secondary to obstruction or the resection is far proximal, a sutured anastomosis is preferable. Both techniques are described here.

Step 3: Operative Steps

1. Stapled Anastomosis

- A window is created between the mesenteric wall of the bowel and the mesentery between vascular arcades with the assistance of cautery and a curved clamp. This is done proximally and distally in an area of viable tissue or with an adequate margin in oncologic resections. (Figure 23-1AB)
- The GIA 60-mm length, 3.8-mm height, linear cutting stapler, is then applied and inserted through the window at a slightly oblique angle. (Figure 23-2AB)

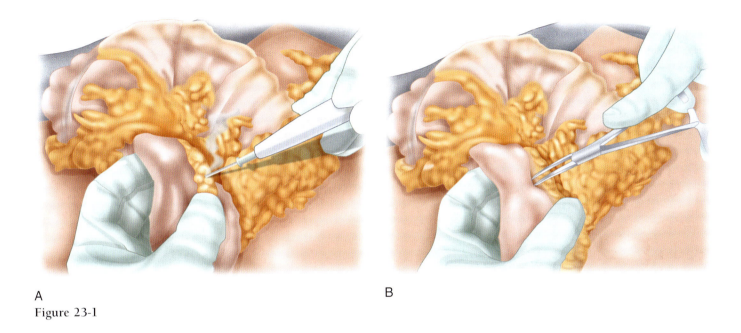

A

Figure 23-1

B

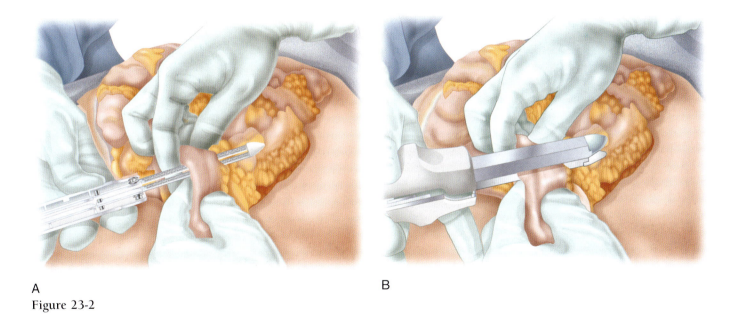

A

Figure 23-2

B

- The linear cutting stapler is fired from the antimesenteric to the mesenteric side to transect the intestine.
- The mesentery is then divided between Kelly clamps. (Figure 23-3AB)
- In oncologic resection the primary vessel supplying the segment is divided at its base to harvest sufficient lymph nodes.
- The vascular supply to the segment is then tied as the clamps are removed and the specimen is handed off the field.
- The two stapled ends are brought in close proximity and aligned in a parallel fashion, and the base of the mesentery is examined to be sure there is no abnormal rotation.
- A towel is brought on the field to prevent any unnecessary spillage of enteric contents into the abdominal cavity.
- Two Alice clamps are placed on the stapled antimesenteric corner of each end; the corner is removed with a curved Mayo scissor; and the clamps are replaced in the lumen of the bowel and applied full thickness to the outer serosa.
- One limb of the GIA 60-mm, 3.8-mm linear cutting stapler, is inserted in each end of the bowel where the enterotomy was made, and the stapler is joined in the intermediate locking position. (Figure 23-4)
- The stapler is closed, and a 3-0 absorbable stitch is placed 1 cm distal to the tip of the stapler as a seromuscular bite in each limb to reduce tension on the corner of the anastomosis.
- The stapler is then fired. (Figure 23-5)
- The two segments are anastomosed with two double-staggered rows of staples.
- An empty sponge stick is inserted through the opening and spread to search for any active bleeding. It is controlled with a 3-0 absorbable suture.
- The remaining enterotomy is closed with a TA 60 or GIA 60 stapler, ensuring that the serosa is incorporated on both sides. (Figure 23-6)
- Two 3-0 polyglactin 910 sutures are placed as Lembert sutures in the corner of the newly fashioned anastomosis and the corners are inverted beneath the tie.

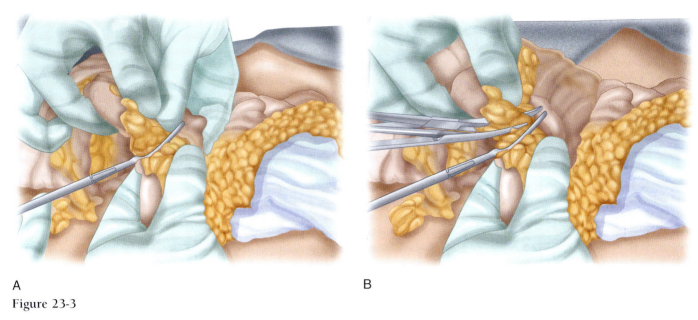

A

B

Figure 23-3

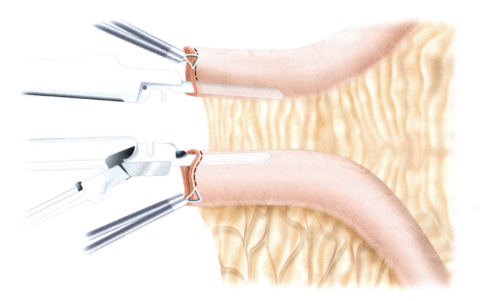

Figure 23-4

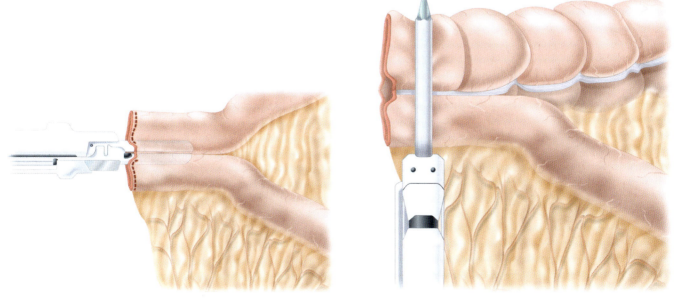

Figure 23-5

Figure 23-6

2. Hand-Sewn Anastomosis

- The segment of small bowel to be resected is placed on a towel to prevent spillage.
- Windows are made in the mesentery parallel to the desired border of small intestine that will be transected. (Figure 23-7AB)
- The mesentery between the windows is divided and tied with Kelly clamps. (Figure 23-8)
- Two curved bowel clamps are placed across the surface of the intestine at the desired location of transaction on each side. (Figure 23-9)
- The bowel is divided with a scalpel, leaving 1 cm of tissue distal to the clamp. (Figure 23-10)

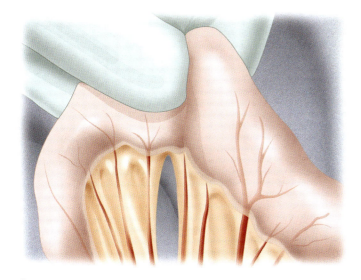

A
Figure 23-7

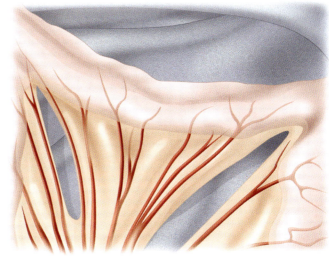

B

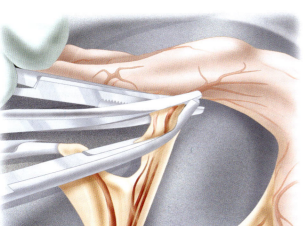
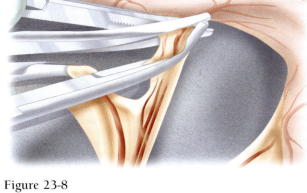

Figure 23-8

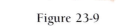

Figure 23-9

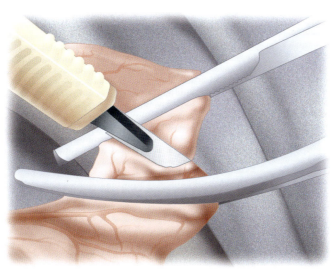

Figure 23-10

- The ends are brought in proximity to one another and two stay sutures are placed, joining the ends. (Figure 23-11ABC)
- A two-layer anastomosis is then performed. (Figure 23-12)

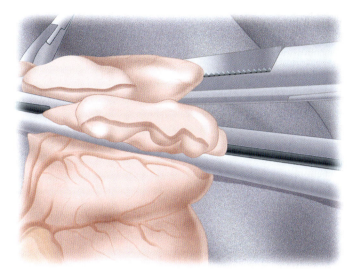

A

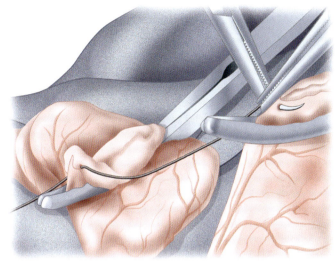

B

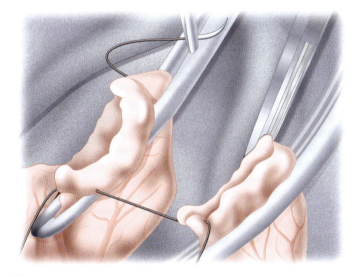

C

Figure 23-11

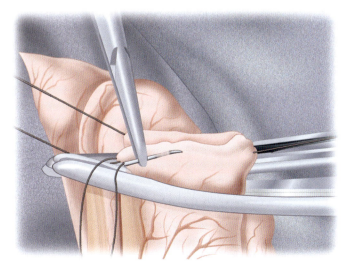

Figure 23-12

◆ The posterior inner layer is performed by starting in the center of the anastomosis, placing two full-thickness sutures through each loop of intestine and tying them together. They are then run continuously until the corner is reached. (Figure 23-13ABC)
◆ When the corner is reached a Connell stitch is performed in the anterior inner layer, and the ends are again tied in the center.
◆ Lembert interrupted sutures are placed in the outer layer anteriorly. (Figure 23-14)

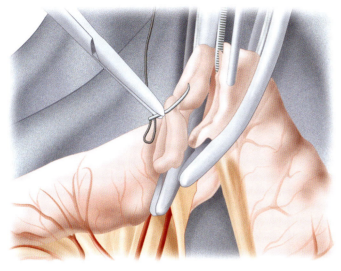

A

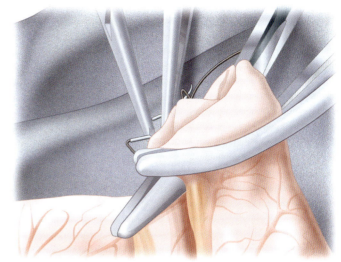

B

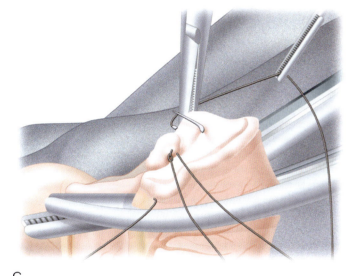

C

Figure 23-13

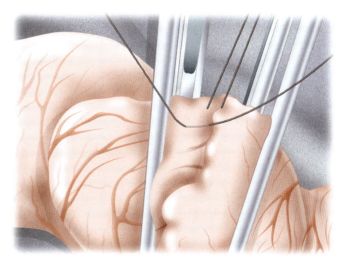

Figure 23-14

- The anastomosis is inverted and the second layer is placed posteriorly again as Lembert sero-muscular interrupted bites. (Figures 23-15AB and 23-16)

Step 4: Postoperative Steps

- Nasogastric tube placement is rarely necessary.
- Beginning oral nutrition is controversial, but likely is not related to postoperative leak rates.

Step 5: Pearls and Pitfalls

- Ensuring excellent blood supply, no tension, and a meticulous surgical technique should minimize chances of anastomotic leaks.
- High-risk anastomosis can be protected by a temporary proximal loop ileostomy/jejunostomy depending on the location of the anastomosis.

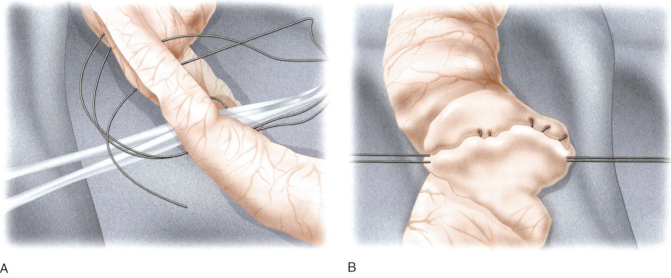

A

B

Figure 23-15

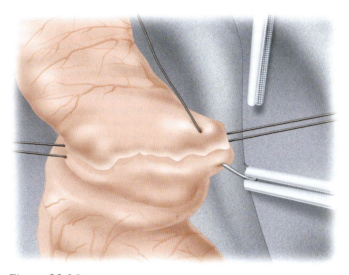

Figure 23-16

CHAPTER 24

JEJUNOSTOMY TUBE

Bradley Champagne, MD

Step 1: Surgical Anatomy

- Identifying the appropriate loop of jejunum approximately 20 cm distal to the duodenojejunal junction is important to achieve maximal nutritional benefits.

Step 2: Preoperative Considerations

- The procedure may be performed under local infiltration or block in patients that will not tolerate general anesthesia, if exploration of the abdomen is not required. If the patient's medical condition allows general anesthesia or the abdomen needs to be explored these approaches are suitable.
- Jejunostomy tubes should typically be reserved for patients with contraindications to a gastrostomy tube, as jejunostomy tubes are associated with a higher morbidity rate.

Step 3: Operative Steps

1. Witzel Technique

- A vertical left paramedian or rectus incision is made. The incision is typically 5 to 6 cm long and begins immediately below the costal margin and one half centimeter posterior to the anterior axillary line. (Figure 24-1A) The incision is carried to the peritoneum through the external oblique, internal oblique, and transversalis muscles. The peritoneum is opened for 3 cm. A high loop of jejunum typically presents itself 20 to 25 cm distal from the duodenojejunal flexure. If this loop is not apparent, the initial part of the jejunum at the duodenojejunal angle is palpated under the transverse colon and mesocolon at the left of the spine. The first bowel loop is gently grasped with a Babcock forcep or finger and withdrawn through the abdominal wound. Ideally, the site selected should be 20 to 40 cm from the duodenojejunal angle.

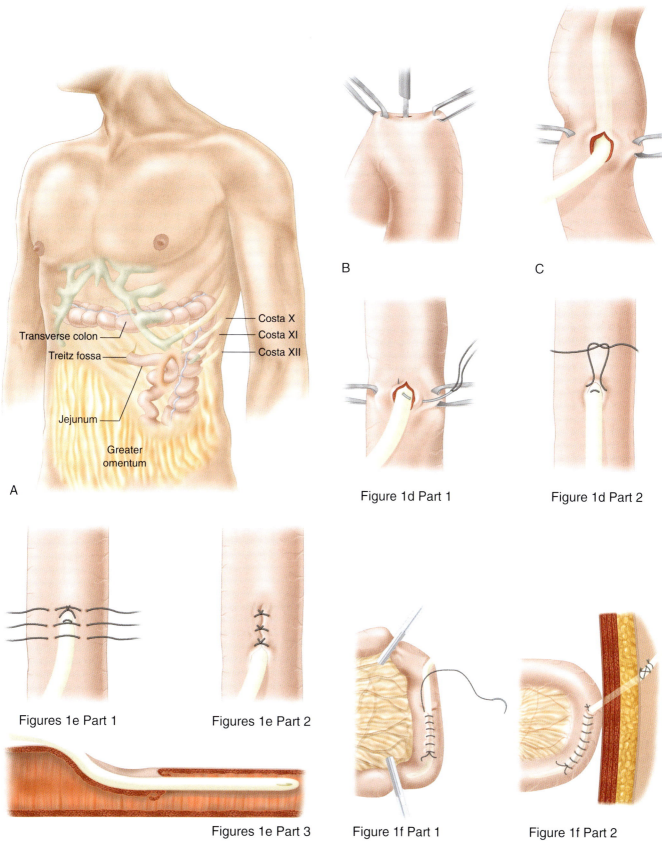

Transverse colon

Costa X
Costa XI
Costa XII

Treitz fossa

Jejunum

Greater omentum

A

B

C

Figure 1d Part 1

Figure 1d Part 2

Figures 1e Part 1

Figures 1e Part 2

Figures 1e Part 3

Figure 1f Part 1

Figure 1f Part 2

Figure 24-1

- An enterotomy is then made in the antimesenteric aspect of the bowel, and the catheter is passed distally at least 7.5 cm into the distal lumen.
- The tube is anchored to the lumen by a single absorbable stitch, which passes through the walls of the intestinal incision and into, not through, the wall of the tube.
- The catheter is then bent back over the bowel and is made to depress the bowel wall slightly, while the outer coats of the intestine are suture-folded over the rubber tube by interrupted seromuscular stitches. This is performed until the tube is completely buried in the jejunal wall. (Figure 24-1BCD, parts 1 and 2) Just enough intestinal wall is used to fit snugly around the tube to prevent significant narrowing of the lumen of the bowel. (Figure 24-1E, parts 1, 2, and 3)
- If there is omentum available, the free end of the tube is passed through the omentum. The omentum is fixed over the suture line with 2 to 3 absorbable sutures. The free end of the catheter is then brought out a separate small stab wound in the abdominal wall. The bowel is then sutured to the abdominal wall over a broad area. (Figure 24-1F, parts 1 and 2)

2. Stamm-Kader Technique

- This procedure is generally reserved for patients who have a distended jejunum or insufficient length for a Witzel.
- An enterotomy is made in exposed jejunum on the antimesenteric side between two concentric purse-string sutures. The first bite of the purse-string should be backhand and the remainder forehand. The first purse-string should be of catgut and should include a bite made tangentially in the wall of the rubber tube. The subsequent purse-string sutures may be of absorbable or nonabsorbable suture, and all should be seromuscular only, not penetrating the lumen.
- The catheter is inserted through the two purse-string sutures.
- The catheter is fixed to the abdominal wall. (Figure 24-2ABCD)
- The catheter is brought out through an opening as described above.

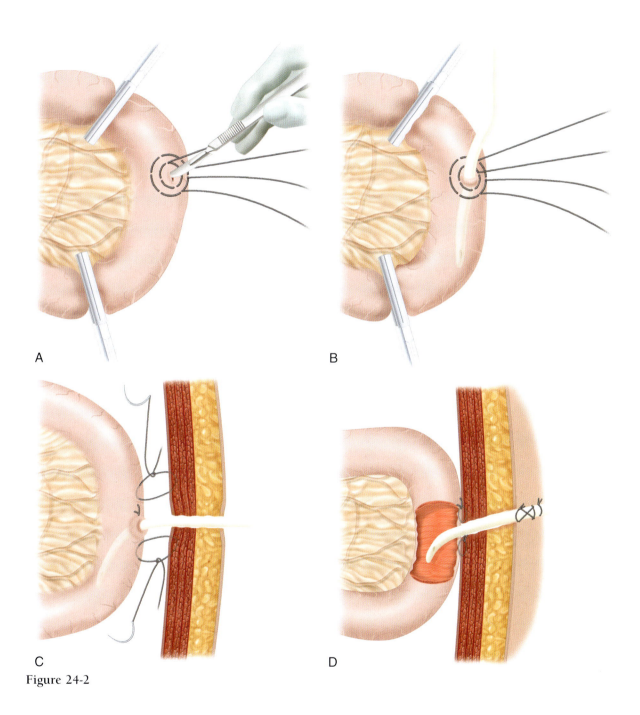

A

B

C

D

Figure 24-2

3. Permanent Technique

- The abdominal cavity can usually be opened through a left paramedian or rectus-splitting incision. The proximal loop of jejunum 20 to 25 cm from the duodenojejunal angle is brought into the wound and transected between clamps.
- The mesentery that parallels this transection line should be divided for 10 cm to increase mobility.
- The distal cut end of the jejunum is brought out through a separate incision lateral to the original incision. Three centimeters of jejunum are left protruding from the skin edge and it is then fixed with eight interrupted absorbable sutures anchoring the bowel wall to the subcuticular layer of skin.
- Through the abdominal incision the cut end of the proximal jejunal segment is anastomosed to the side of the distal segment at a point at least 45 cm distal to the jejunostomy stoma. (Figure 24-3)

Step 4: Postoperative Steps

- Tubes should be flushed with 10 cc of saline each shift, and after each feeding to avoid clogging. Tube feeding is typically started 24 hours after placement.

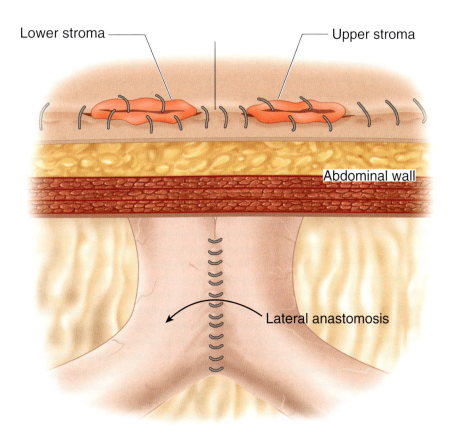

Figure 24-3

Step 5: Pearls and Pitfalls

- Unlike a gastrostomy tube that maintains the wide mesentery of the stomach, a jejunostomy tube is prone to volvulus. The jejunum therefore should be secured over a broad area of the abdominal wall to minimize the chances of volvulus.
- Since most of the tubes are Witzeled, if a jejunostomy tube becomes dislodged it should be replaced fairly quickly to avoid loss of the track. If the track cannot be obtained, using fluoroscopy and guide wires can often salvage these tubes.
- Whenever replacing a tube, a tube injection study should be performed with diluted contrast material to confirm appropriate placement of the catheter prior to feeding.
- The Witzel method should be avoided in the setting of distended or obstructed bowel because the seromuscular sutures through a paper-thin bowel wall cannot be made without entering the lumen.

CHAPTER 25

STRICTUREPLASTY FOR CROHN'S DISEASE

Bradley Champagne, MD

Step 1: Surgical Anatomy

- Complex patients with Crohn disease should undergo a small bowel follow-through to delineate the extent of their disease and the amount of small bowel they may be left with. Upper and lower endoscopy are also helpful to evaluate other sites of disease and guide operative planning.

Step 2: Preoperative Considerations

- With advancements in the medical and surgical management of Crohn disease, resection is the most common surgical procedure. However, a small percentage of patients with extensive strictures or who are at risk of short bowel or who have short bowel syndrome may require strictureplasty. The two procedures described here are for short and long segments involved with stricture. These techniques are associated with low anastomotic leak rates and complications.

Step 3: Operative Steps

1. Heineke-Mikulicz (Short <8 cm)

- Carefully inspect the entire intestine to develop a strategy. Measure the remaining small bowel and record the length of strictures in the medical record. If unsure about the need for strictureplasty, the 2 cm required for bowel lumen can be tested by passing a Foley through another site and inflating to 6 cc which is 2 cm.

- The bowel above and below the proposed strictureplasty site is isolated with Satinsky clamps to prevent spillage. Using the cutting cautery, the seromuscular layer is incised down to the submucosal level. The incision is made 3 cm proximal and distal to the stricture to reach healthy bowel. (Figure 25-1)
- An enterotomy is made over the nonstrictured bowel end, and angled forceps are used to spread the enterotomy.
- Exposed submucosa and mucosa of the anterior wall of the stricture are then divided.
- Seromuscular sutures of 3-0 polyglactin 910 are placed opposite one another at the midpoint of the defect and separated with clamps. (Figure 25-2)
- The mucosa is then biopsied.
- Lateral traction is applied, and the longitudinal defect is converted to a transverse defect. (Figure 25-3)
- Single-layer interrupted extramucosal layer is performed with 3-0 sutures at 2 mm intervals, and a radiographic clip is applied. (Figure 25-4)

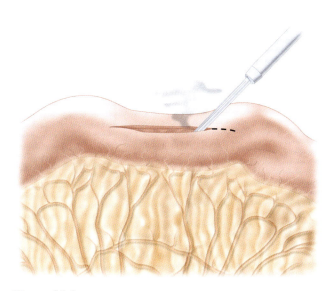

Figure 25-1

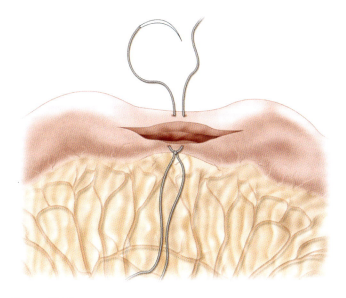

Figure 25-2

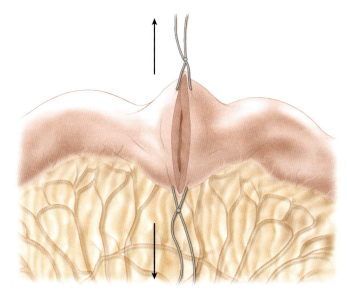

Figure 25-3

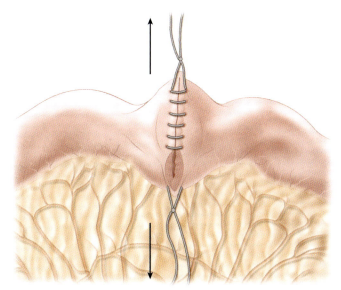

Figure 25-4

2. Finney (Long)

- An enterotomy similar to that previously described for short strictureplasty is used but is made anterolaterally. (Figure 25-5)
- The open segment is then folded in half onto itself.
- The tight strictured segment is aligned against a relatively normal caliber segment.
- A continuous 2-0 Vicryl suture joins the medial edges of the defect. Sutures are placed through all layers of the bowel edge. (Figure 25-6)
- This layer is then reinforced with interrupted 3-0 Vicryl to further approximate any nonopposed mucosa where possible. (Figure 25-7)
- The anterior layer is then closed with interrupted 2-0 Vicryl in one layer using seromuscular sutures.

Step 4: Postoperative Steps

- None.

Step 5: Pearls and Pitfalls

- Contraindications to performing a strictureplasty include perforation, fistula, or ischemia at the site. Furthermore, performing this procedure in close proximity to another resection of strictureplasty is not recommended.

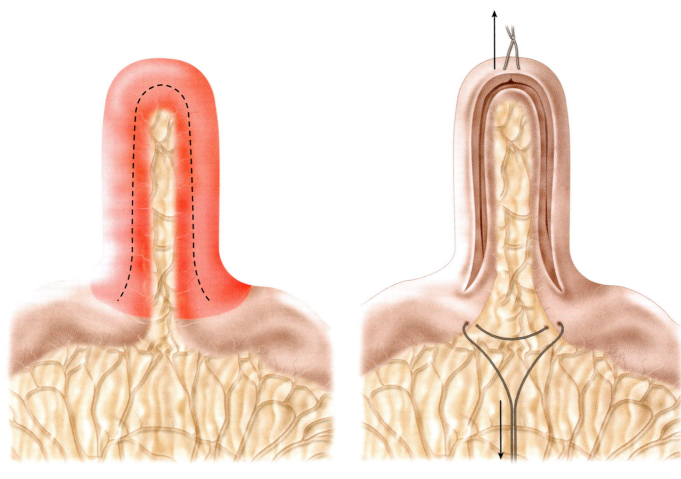

Figure 25-5

Figure 25-6

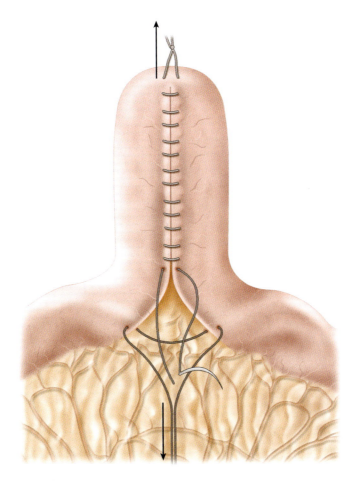

Figure 25-7

CHAPTER 26

LAPAROSCOPY FOR CROHN'S DISEASE

Bradley Champagne, MD

Step 1: Surgical Anatomy

- None.

Step 2: Preoperative Considerations

- The most common laparoscopic resection for Crohn disease is unquestionably ileocecal resection. The conduct and intraoperative steps vary depending on presentation and intraoperative findings. The medial to lateral approach described below is typically used with two notable exceptions:
  - ▲ Thickened mesentery. If the mesentery is very bulky and difficult to handle laparoscopically, bleeding can be profuse when attempting to divide the ileocolic pedicle. In these cases the entire mobilization is performed, but the vascular pedicle is safely taken extracorporeally.
  - ▲ Mesenteric phlegmon/abscess. In the setting where the mesentery is occupied by a large abscess or phlegmon a lateral to medial approach is appropriate.

Step 3: Operative Steps

1. Routine Ileocecal Resection

- Patient positioning: All patients are positioned with yellowfin stirrups with the legs parallel to the bed and the arms tucked. (Figure 26-1AB)
- The primary monitor is placed on the right side of the patient. (Figure 26-2)
- An umbilical port is placed with an open Hasson technique, and a 10-mm, 30-degree camera is inserted.

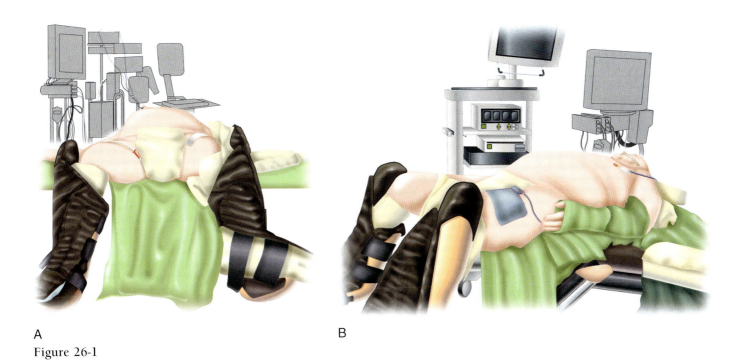

A

B

Figure 26-1

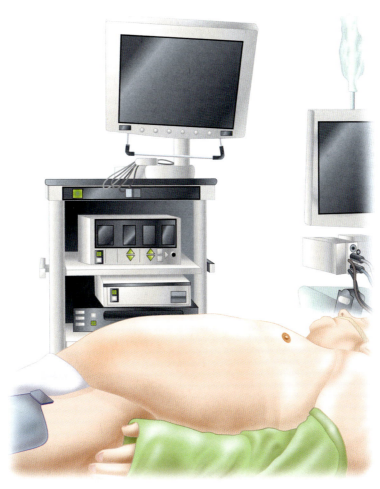

Figure 26-2

- Additional ports: A 5-mm port is inserted 2 fingerbreadths medial to and 3 fingerbreadths superior to the right anterior superior iliac spine. Another 5-mm port is inserted in the left upper quadrant. Abdominal exploration is performed, and the small intestine is run from the ligament of Treitz to the cecum, noting any strictures or fistulas. (Figure 26-3)
- If the mesentery is approachable and not involved with disease, a 12-mm port is inserted in the lower left quadrant. All ports are inserted lateral to the epigastric vessels.
- The assistant moves to the left side and holds the camera and right lower quadrant port. The surgeon works through the two left-sided ports. (Figure 26-4)
- The table is placed in a slight Trendelenburg position and tilted to the left.
- The omentum is reflected cephalad so that it lies on the stomach, and the small bowel is moved to the patient's left side to allow visualization of the ileocolic pedicle.
- A noncrushing bowel clamp is placed on the mesentery at the ileocecal junction to stretch the ileocolic pedicle. (Figure 26-5)
- Scissor cautery is used to open the peritoneum along a line parallel with the vessel. (Figure 26-6)

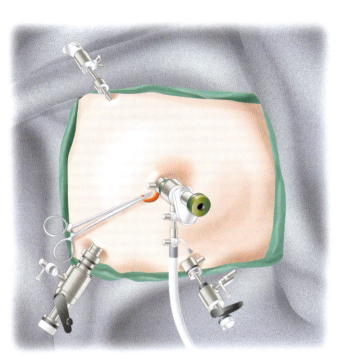

Figure 26-3

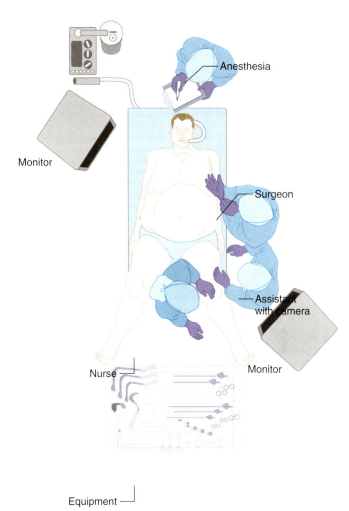

Figure 26-4

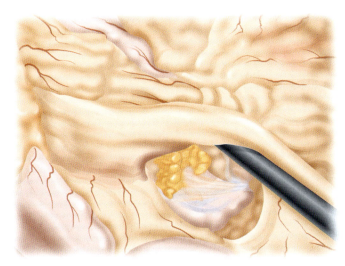

Figure 26-5

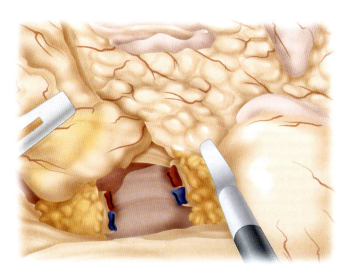

Figure 26-6

- Blunt dissection then is used to lift the vessel off the retroperitoneum and duodenum, and the duodenum is dissected posteriorly. (Figure 26-7)
- The vessel is safely divided after a window is created cephalad with a vascular stapler or bipolar vessel sealer.
- The plane between the ascending colon mesentery and retroperitoneum is bluntly developed until the liver is seen beneath the mesentery. (Figure 26-8)
- The lesser sac is opened, and the hepatic flexure is mobilized.
- The terminal ileum is lifted off of the retroperitoneal, and the ascending colon is mobilized.
- The specimen is extracted via a 3- to 4-cm periumbilical incision. (Figure 26-9AB)
- Resection and anastomosis are performed as described in Chapter 23.
- The midline wound is closed.
- Pneumoperitoneum is reestablished and the left lower quadrant port is closed with the aid of a 5-mm camera. (Figure 26-10)

Step 4: Postoperative Steps

- None.

Step 5: Pearls and Pitfalls

- The intense inflammatory reaction and often foreshortened mesentery can make laparoscopic resection for Crohn disease treacherous. These procedures should only be attempted after extensive experience with laparoscopic colectomy for other indications.

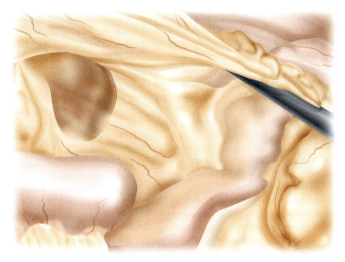

Figure 26-7

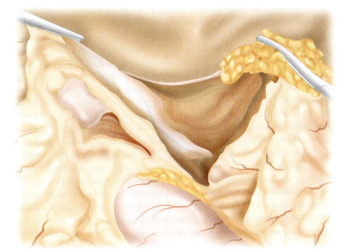

Figure 26-8

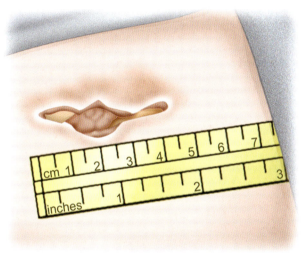

A

Figure 26-9

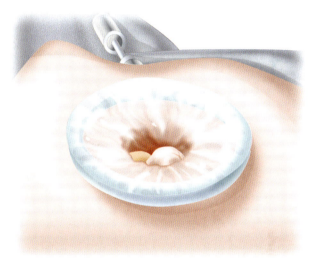

B

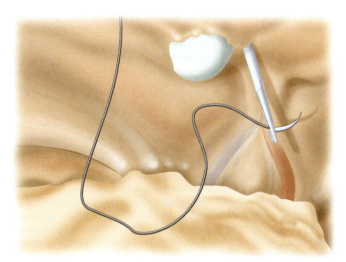

Figure 26-10

CHAPTER 27

MECKEL DIVERTICULECTOMY

Bradley Champagne, MD

Step 1: Surgical Anatomy

- Meckel diverticulum is a congenital diverticulum that is a result of a remnant omphalomesenteric duct. It is typically located 2 feet from the ileocecal valve, and is present in 2% of the population.
- Meckel diverticulum can contain ectopic pancreatic and gastric mucosa that can predispose to mucosal ulcerations, bleeding, infection, obstruction, and perforations.

Step 2: Preoperative Considerations

- Operative management of the Meckel diverticulum depends on the indications for surgery, the intraoperative findings, and surgeon's preference. The two options that exist are wide excision of the diverticulum or intestinal resection.
- In the setting of intussusception with the Meckel diverticulum as the lead point, wide excision is acceptable. For bleeding, intestinal resection is preferred because the ulceration is typically on the mesenteric side of the bowel opposite the diverticulum. The resection and anastomosis is identical for that of a hand-sewn small bowel resection described in Chapter 23, Small Bowel Resection and Anastomosis.
- Incidentally found Meckel diverticulums typically do not require resection.

Step 3: Operative Steps

- The open approach is performed through a transverse right lower quadrant incision. (Figure 27-1)
- The cecum is identified, and the terminal ileum is pulled into the wound and examined proximally until the Meckel diverticulum is reached.
- Excision is performed as follows:
  - ▲ A longitudinally oriented enterotomy around the base of the diverticulum is performed with needlepoint monopoloar cautery. (Figure 27-2)

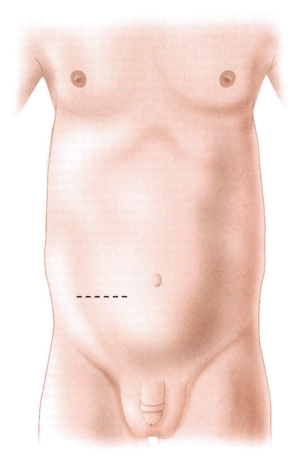

Figure 27-1

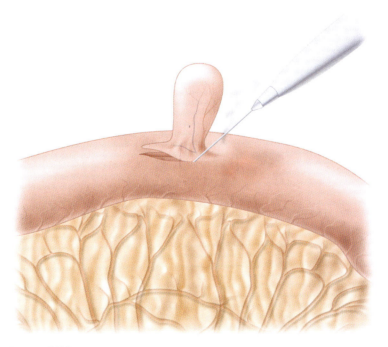

Figure 27-2

▲ The Meckel diverticulum is removed.
▲ The excision is closed in a transverse fashion.
▲ A continuous Connell suture is started outside the bowel, done in one layer. (Figure 27-3)
▲ This decreases the chance of diminishing the lumen size. (Figure 27-4)
▲ In recent years, stapling as depicted in Figures 27-5 and 27-6 has also become popular and is performed with a TA or GIA cartridge. (Figures 27-5 and 27-6 parts 1 and 2)

Step 4: Postoperative Steps

♦ None.

Step 5: Pearls and Pitfalls

♦ In cases of gastrointestinal bleeding from unidentified sources, one should always consider a Meckel diverticulum.
♦ A segmental resection is appropriate in cases of bleeding, to resect the bleeding ulcer opposite the Meckel diverticulum.

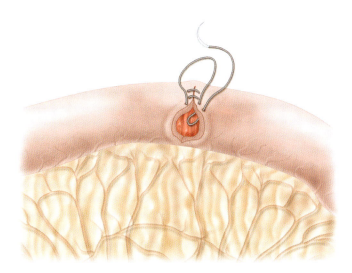

Figure 27-3

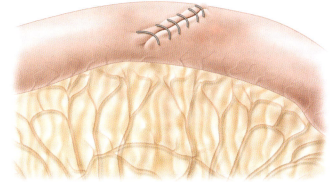

Figure 27-4

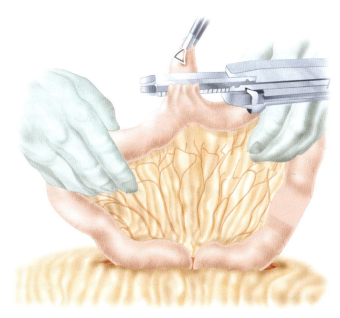

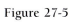

Figure 27-5

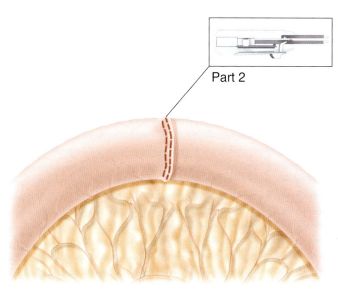

Part 2

Part 1
Figure 27-6

CHAPTER 28

Intussception Eduction

Bradley Champagne, MD

Step 1: Surgical Anatomy

- Intussception can occur at any age, but only 10% occur after the age of 2. All intussceptions in the adult population need to be managed by segmental resection, and the technique is described in Chapter 23, Small Bowel Resection and Anastomosis.

Step 2: Preoperative Considerations

- Nonoperative Management: Once the diagnosis of intussception is made and resuscitation is initiated, hydrostatic or pneumatic reduction can be considered in the absence of peritonitis, perforation, advanced sepsis, or gangrenous bowel. This decision is made by the surgeon. These techniques have been successful in 75% to 94% of cases. After the procedure the patient should be observed NPO for 24 hours.
- Operative Management: Indicated in children with signs of shock, peritonitis, or incomplete reduction. Antibiotics, nasogastric tube decompression, and intravenous fluids are given preoperatively.

Step 3: Operative Steps

- A right lower quadrant transverse muscle-splitting incision or lower midline incision is appropriate. The incision can be extended if required. (Figure 28-1)
- Identify the intussception, typically the terminal ileum into the right colon. The right colon should be delivered into the wound as much as possible. (Figure 28-2)
- Assessment: If a necrotic bowel is identified, resection is indicated.
- Gentle manipulation of the bowel with "pushing," not pulling the lead point to its normal position is initiated. Very little to no traction should be placed on the ileum. (Figure 28-3)
- If resistance occurs and serosal tears are imminent, further attempts may lead to perforation. Contamination and resection is warranted. (Figure 28-4)

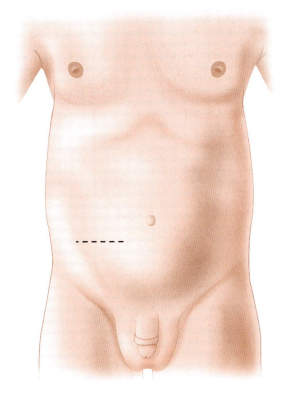

Figure 28-1

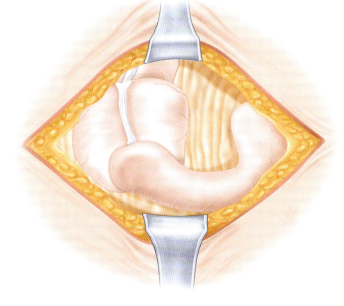

Figure 28-2

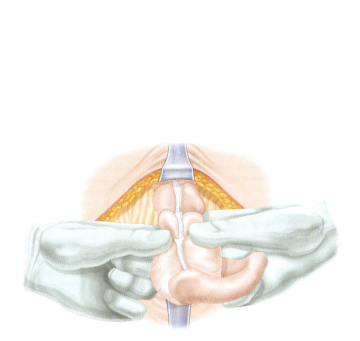

Figure 28-3

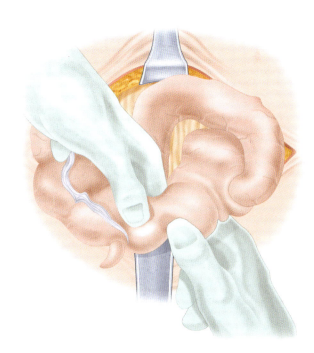

Figure 28-4

- After complete reduction, warm packs are applied to the bowel and viability is addressed.
- A lead point is sought. Typically umbilicated Peyer patches on terminal ileum or a Meckel diverticulum are the cause in adults. If a Meckel diverticulum is identified, it should be resected.
- An appendectomy is typically performed to eliminate future diagnostic dilemmas.

Step 4: Postoperative Steps

- Recurrence of intussception postoperatively can occur. In patients with excessive or recurrent abdominal pain, consideration of reexploration should be given.

Step 5: Pearls and Pitfalls

- In adults with intussception, tumors can serve as the lead point, and if suspected an appropriate oncologic resection should be performed.
- If perforation occurs intraoperatively or preoperatively, or if gangrenous bowel is identified, an ileocecal resection should be carried out.
- Laparoscopy can be performed but only by those with extensive experience in laparoscopy in children. The approach offers very little to the operation because the intusceptum requires manual reduction.
- In cases with questionable bowel viability, a planned second-look procedure is appropriate.

SMALL BOWEL OBSTRUCTION

Bradley Champagne, MD

Step 1: Surgical Anatomy

- None.

Step 2: Preoperative Considerations

- Patients with small bowel obstructions require careful preoperative evaluation. Neither history, physical exam, nor laboratory evaluation have proven reliable in determining impending ischemia to the intestines. Therefore, a high index of suspicion for operative intervention, especially in complete obstructions, is warranted.
- Plain abdominal films, CT scans, and small bowel follow-throughs are all useful adjuncts in determining whether the obstruction is complete or partial.
- Volume shifts and electrolyte abnormalities can be significant in high-grade small bowel obstructions and should be carefully assessed preoperatively.

Step 3: Operative Steps

1. Open Resection

- When the decision to operate for small bowel resection has been made, it is critical to communicate the condition of the patient and diagnosis with the anesthesiologist to ensure that all precautions against aspiration are performed.
- Incision: The choice is crucial. A midline laparotomy is typically preferred but should be extended to an area of virgin abdomen to minimize the risk of bowel injury. In some cases a transverse incision at or above the umbilicus can be considered.
- The abdomen cavity is entered without cautery; a scalpel or pair of scissors is preferred.

- Free adhesions along the length of the wound with a Kocher clamp on the fascia and tension and counter tension on the adhesions. (Figure 29-1)
- Observe the character of the peritoneal fluid and take cultures.
- Sharp dissection of adhesions and identify transition point. (Figure 29-2)
- If a transition point is readily identified and the remaining small intestine proximally is dilated and distally is decompressed, the adhesions at this location can be divided and no further dissection is needed. (Figure 29-3)
- If unclear or multiple segments of dilated and decompressed bowel, lysing all adhesions from ligament of Treitz to cecum is essential.
- If adhesions are too dense to delineate the appropriate plane, inject adhesions with saline. (Figure 29-4)
- Assess viability; consider resection.
- Bypass: If a dilated loop is entering the pelvis, a clear decompressed loop is emerging, and the pelvis is hostile with a history of radiation or sepsis, an intestinal bypass can be considered. It is performed as a hand-sewn, side-to-side anastomosis as pictured in two layers, similar to that in Chapter 23.
- Repair enterotomies with interrupted 3-0 absorbable suture.
- Decompress intestinal contents by milking into duodenum with a nasogastric tube.
- Close fascia and skin unless gangrenous bowel is present or there is severe contamination.

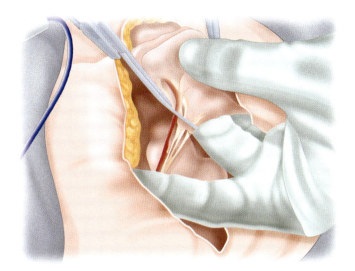

Figure 29-1

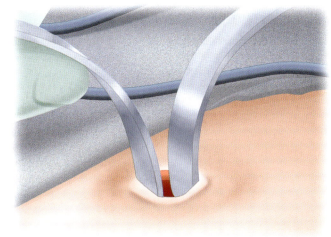

Figure 29-2

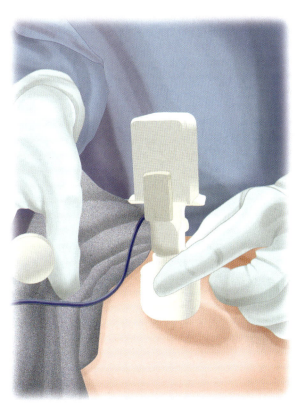

Figure 29-3

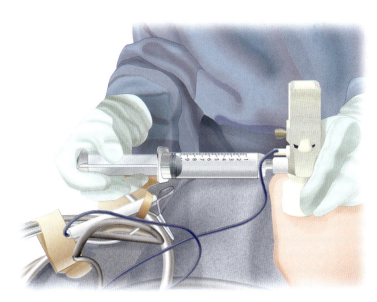

Figure 29-4

2. Laparoscopy

◆ Indications: Similar to those for open surgery, but patients with sepsis or evidence of perforation or necrosis should not be included.
◆ Obtaining pneumoperitoneum: Typically an open Hasson technique is used via a 10-mm incision in the right or left upper quadrant, depending on previous surgery. If previous pathology was on the left, enter on the right; if previous surgery was on the right, enter on the left. For patients with previous pelvic surgery only, hysterectomy etc., an upper midline trocar will suffice.
◆ After the incision is made, S retractors are used, and the anterior fascia is incised. (Figure 29-5) The muscle is retracted, and the posterior fascia and peritoneum are dissected sharply. The abdomen is entered sharply. A balloon port is then placed. (Figures 29-6 and 29-7)
◆ Additional 5-mm ports are then placed depending on intraabdominal findings. Ideally they are placed parallel to the camera.
◆ Anterior abdominal adhesions should be divided without monopolar or bipolar cautery.
◆ Atraumatic bowel graspers are used to identify the transition point.
◆ Adhesiolysis is completed in this region.

Step 4: Postoperative Steps

◆ A nasogastric tube is typically left in place for several days after surgery, as the distension of the bowel can result in a prolonged ileus.

Step 5: Pearls and Pitfalls

◆ When exploring the abdomen in the setting of a small bowel obstruction, with dilated intestines, whether open or laparoscopically, the surgeon should avoid handling the dilated bowel. Begin at the ileocecal valve, and run backwards to the transition point.

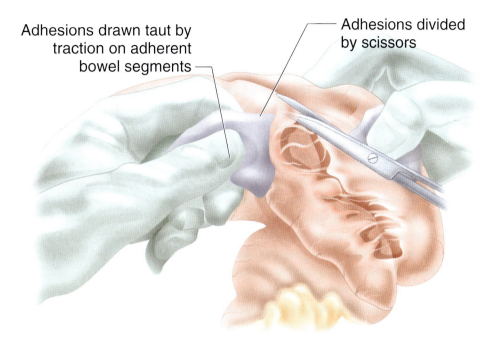

Adhesions drawn taut by traction on adherent bowel segments

Adhesions divided by scissors

Figure 29-5

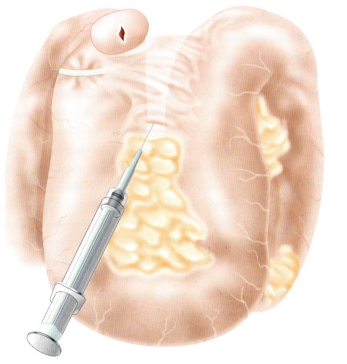

Figure 29-6

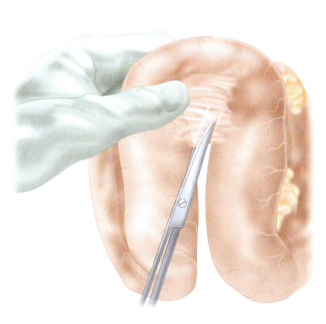

Figure 29-7

INDEX

Page numbers followed by f indicate figures

A

Achalasia
  botulinum injection in, 65, 70
  cause of, 65
  Heller myotomy in, 65–71
  pneumatic dilatation in, 65, 70
Adhesions, small bowel obstruction in, 232, 234
Afferent loop syndrome, postgastrectomy, 134, 135f
Alkaline reflux, postgastrectomy, 132, 133f
  gastritis in, 150f
Ampulla of Vater in antrectomy, identification of, 118
Anastomosis
  in antrectomy, 114, 115f, 118, 119f, 120, 121f
    with Billroth II reconstruction, 120, 122
    hand-sewn, 114
    stapled, 122
  in esophagectomy
    Ivor Lewis, 15, 18, 19f, 20
    left thoracoabdominal, 21, 22, 24, 25f
    minimally invasive, 33, 38
    transhiatal, 30
    tri-incisional, 2, 10
  in gastrectomy
    subtotal, 151f, 152
    total, 154, 156f, 157f–159f, 160
  in gastric bypass, Roux-en-Y
    in jejunojejunostomy creation, 164–166, 165f, 167f
    leaks at, 174
  in small bowel resection, 194–205
    hand-sewn, 194, 198–204, 199f, 201f, 203f, 205f
    leaks at, 204
    in obstruction, 232
    stapled, 194–196, 195f, 197f
"Angle of sorrow" in antrectomy, 118
Antibiotics, preoperative
  in Finney pyloroplasty, 97
  in gastric bypass, Roux-en-Y, 162
  in gastric sleeve, 188
  in Heineke-Mikulicz pyloroplasty, 88
  in tri-incisional esophagectomy, 1
Antiemetics, postoperative
  in Nissen fundoplication, 50
  in paraesophageal hernia repair, 62
Antireflux procedures
  in Heller myotomy, 68–70
  in paraesophageal hernia repair, 60
Antrectomy, 110–126
  Billroth I reconstruction in, 110, 112, 116, 124
  Billroth II reconstruction in, 120, 122
  contraindications to, 110, 112
  dumping syndrome in, 127, 128, 129f
  indications for, 110
  operative steps in, 112–124
    anastomosis in, 114, 115f, 118, 119f, 120, 121f, 122
    angle of sorrow in, 118
    closure, 124, 125f, 126
    dissection, 112–124
    incision, 112
  pearls and pitfalls in, 126
  postoperative care in, 124, 126
  preoperative considerations in, 110
  pyloroplasty compared to, 87
  Roux stasis syndrome in, 134, 135f
  surgical anatomy in, 110, 111f
  vagotomy with, 72, 86, 87, 110
    alkaline reflux in, 132, 133f
    anatomy in, 111f
    dumping syndrome in, 128, 129f
    gastroparesis in, 130, 131f

Antrectomy (Continued)
    laparoscopic, 137
    operative steps in, 112, 114
Antrum, gastric
  in Jaboulay pyloroplasty, 104, 106
  resection of, 110–126
  tumors of, 149f
Aorta
  in antrectomy, 111f
  in esophagectomy, left thoracoabdominal, 21, 24, 26
  in paraesophageal hernia repair, 58, 59f
Appendiceal retractors in gastric banding, 184, 186
Arrhythmias, postoperative
  in gastric bypass, 174
  in tri-incisional esophagectomy, 12
Aspiration pneumonia in tri-incisional esophagectomy, 12
Atrial fibrillation in tri-incisional esophagectomy, 12
Azygous vein in esophagectomy
  Ivor Lewis, 15, 17
  thoracoscopic, 34
  transhiatal, 30, 32
  tri-incisional, 1, 2, 3f, 4, 13

B

Band, gastric, 177–186. See also Gastric banding, laparoscopic.
Bariatric surgery, 161–193
  gastric band in, 177–186
  gastric bypass in, Roux-en-Y, 161–176
  gastric sleeve in, 187–193
Bile reflux, postgastrectomy, 132, 133f
  gastritis in, 150f
Billroth I reconstruction
  alkaline reflux in, 132, 133f
    and gastritis in, 150f
  in antrectomy, 110, 112, 116, 124
  dumping syndrome in, 128, 129f
Billroth II reconstruction
  in afferent or efferent loop syndrome, postgastrectomy, 134, 135f
  alkaline reflux in, 132, 133f
    and gastritis in, 150f
  in antrectomy, 120, 122
  dumping syndrome in, 128, 129f
  in gastroparesis, postgastrectomy, 130, 131f
Blake drains in esophagectomy
  in Ivor Lewis technique, 18, 20
  left thoracoabdominal, 26
Body mass index in bariatric surgery
  in gastric banding, 177, 180
  in gastric bypass, 161
  in gastric sleeve, 187, 192
Botulinum toxin injection in achalasia, 65, 70
Bowel preparation, preoperative
  in Roux-en-Y gastric bypass, 162, 174
  in sleeve gastrectomy, 188
  in tri-incisional esophagectomy, 1
Braun enteroenterostomy in postgastrectomy syndromes
  in gastroparesis, 130, 131f
  in Roux stasis syndrome, 134, 135f
Bypass, gastric Roux-en-Y, 161–176. See also Gastric bypass, Roux-en-Y.

C

Cardiac evaluation in esophagectomy, preoperative, 1
Celiac artery in antrectomy, 111f

Celiac lymph node dissection in tri-incisional esophagectomy, 6
Cervical incisions
  in transhiatal esophagectomy, 28, 29f
  in tri-incisional esophagectomy, 8, 10, 11f
Chest tubes
  in Ivor Lewis esophagectomy, 18
  in transhiatal esophagectomy, 32
  in tri-incisional esophagectomy, 4, 12
Chyle leaks
  in minimally invasive esophagectomy, 39
  in tri-incisional esophagectomy, 12
Colic arteries in antrectomy, 112, 113f
Compression devices in thromboembolism prevention, 1, 12
Connell stitch
  in antrectomy, 118, 122
  in Meckel diverticulectomy, 226
  in small bowel resection and anastomosis, 202
Costal margin
  in esophagectomy, left thoracoabdominal, incision across, 22, 24, 26
  in gastric bypass port placement, 162
  in gastric sleeve port placement, 188
  in paraesophageal hernia repair port placement, 55
  in Witzel jejunostomy incision, 206
Criminal nerve of Grassi
  in selective vagotomy, 79f, 80
  in truncal vagotomy, 73f, 76
Crohn's disease, 213–223
  laparoscopic resection in, 218–223
  strictureplasty in, 213–217
Crus of diaphragm
  in gastric banding, laparoscopic, 177, 180
  in Heller myotomy, 67f
    in Dor fundoplication, 70, 71f
  in Nissen fundoplication
    closure of, 46, 47f, 51
    left crus in, 44, 46, 47f
    right crus in, 42, 43f, 47f
  in paraesophageal hernia repair, 62
    closure of, 60, 61f
    left crus in, 58, 59f, 62
    right crus in, 56, 57f, 58, 59f

D

Deaver retractors
  in esophagectomy, transhiatal, 28
  in gastric banding, 184, 186
DeBakey grasper in gastric banding, 182
Diabetes mellitus
  Roux-en-Y gastric bypass in, 172
  sleeve gastrectomy in, 192
Diaphragm
  in antrectomy, 115f
  crus of. See Crus of diaphragm.
  in esophagectomy
    Ivor Lewis, 16
    left thoracoabdominal, 22, 24, 26
    tri-incisional, 6
Diverticulectomy, Meckel, 224–227
Dor fundoplication in Heller myotomy, 66, 70, 71f
Dumping syndrome, postgastrectomy, 127–128, 129f
Duodenostomy in antrectomy, 126
Duodenum
  in antrectomy, 115f, 126
    assessing quality of, 112, 126

237

Duodenum (*Continued*)
  with Billroth II reconstruction, 122
  closure of, 124, 126
  division of, 116, 118
  mobilization of, 112, 113f, 114, 116, 124
  surgical anatomy of, 110, 111f
  in esophagectomy, tri-incisional, 6
  in Finney pyloroplasty, 98, 99f
    mobilization of, 103
  in gastrectomy, subtotal, 149f
  in Heineke-Mikulicz pyloroplasty, 89f, 92, 93f
    mobilization of, 87, 88
  in Jaboulay pyloroplasty, 104, 109
    mobilization of, 106
  ulcer disease of
    antrectomy in, 110, 118, 124
    Finney pyloroplasty in, 103
    Heineke-Mikulicz pyloroplasty in, 87, 92, 93f
    highly selective vagotomy in, 82
    Jaboulay pyloroplasty and truncal vagotomy in, 104
Dysphagia, postoperative, in Nissen fundoplication, 51

E
Education of patients in bariatric surgery
  in gastric banding, 177, 186
  in gastric bypass, 161, 174
  in gastric sleeve, 187
EEA stapler
  in esophagojejunostomy, 157f–158f
  in gastric bypass, 168, 170, 171f
  in Ivor Lewis esophagectomy, 18
Efferent loop syndrome, postgastrectomy, 134, 135f
Endoscopy
  in gastrectomy
    and postgastrectomy syndromes, 127, 132
    subtotal, 146
    total, 153, 154
  in Heineke-Mikulicz pyloroplasty, preoperative, 87
  in Heller myotomy
    intraoperative, 68
    preoperative, 65
  in paraesophageal hernia repair, preoperative, 55
Endotracheal intubation in total gastrectomy, 153
Enterotomy
  in gastric bypass, 166, 170, 174
  in Meckel diverticulectomy, 224
  in Stamm-Kader jejunostomy, 208
  in strictureplasty for Crohn's disease, 214, 216
  in Witzel jejunostomy, 208
Epidural anesthesia in tri-incisional esophagectomy, 2, 12
Epinephrine injection in Heller myotomy, 66, 67f
Esophagectomy, 1–39
  distal, in total gastrectomy, 153
  Ivor Lewis, 15–20
  left thoracoabdominal, 21–26
  minimally invasive, 33–39
  transhiatal, 27–32
  tri-incisional, 1–13
Esophagogastroduodenoscopy, preoperative, in tri-
    incisional esophagectomy, 2
Esophagojejunostomy, Roux-en-Y, in total gastrectomy,
    157f–159f
Esophagus, 1–39
  in gastrectomy, total
    access to, 154
    operative steps involving, 155f, 156f, 157f–159f, 160
    preoperative evaluation of, 153
    surgical anatomy of, 153
  Heller myotomy of, 65–71
  motility studies of
    in Heller myotomy, 65
    in paraesophageal hernia repair, 55
  in Nissen fundoplication, length of, 46, 50
  in paraesophageal hernia repair
    inadvertent injury of, 56
    length of, 58, 60, 63
    mediastinal mobilization of, 58, 59f, 63
  perforation in Heller myotomy, 70

Esophagus, (*Continued*)
  resection of, 1–39. *See also* Esophagectomy.
  surgical anatomy of
    in Heller myotomy, 65
    in Ivor Lewis esophagectomy, 15
    in left thoracoabdominal approach, 21
    in minimally invasive esophagectomy, 33
    in total gastrectomy, 153
    in transhiatal esophagectomy, 27
    in tri-incisional esophagectomy, 1
Ewald tube, in pouch creation for Roux-en-Y gastric
    bypass, 170, 176

F
Falciform ligament
  division of
    in antrectomy, 112
    in Finney pyloroplasty, 98
    in Heineke-Mikulicz pyloroplasty, 88
    in Jaboulay pyloroplasty, 106
  in port placement
    in gastric banding, 178
    in paraesophageal hernia repair, 55
Finney pyloroplasty, 97–103
  compared to Heineke-Mikulicz pyloroplasty, 97, 98,
    103
  delayed gastric emptying after, 102
  indications for, 97, 103
  operative steps in, 98–100, 99f, 101f
    closure, 100, 101f, 103
    dissection, 98–100, 99f, 101f
    in emergent setting, 98
    incision, 98, 99f
  pearls and pitfalls in, 103
  postoperative care in, 102
  preoperative considerations in, 97
  surgical anatomy in, 97
  suture line leaks in, 102
Finney strictureplasty in Crohn's disease, 216, 217f
Fundoplication
  Dor, in Heller myotomy, 66, 70, 71f
  Nissen, 40–51. *See also* Nissen fundoplication.
  in paraesophageal hernia repair, 60
  Toupet
    in Heller myotomy, 66, 68, 69f
    in paraesophageal hernia, 60

G
Gallbladder in antrectomy, 115f
Gambee stitch in Heineke-Mikulicz pyloroplasty, 90, 91f
Gastrectomy, 145–160
  in esophagectomy, left thoracoabdominal, 21
  postgastrectomy syndromes in, 127–135
  sleeve, 187–193
  subtotal, 145–152
  total, 153–160
Gastric arteries
  in antrectomy, 111f, 112, 116
  in esophagectomy
    laparoscopic, 36
    left thoracoabdominal, 22, 24
    tri-incisional, 6, 8, 13
  in gastrectomy
    subtotal, 145, 147f, 148f, 152
    total, 156f
  in gastric bypass, 164
  in Heller myotomy, 66
  in Nissen fundoplication, 42–44, 43f, 44, 45f, 50
  in paraesophageal hernia repair, 58
Gastric banding, laparoscopic, 177–186
  operative steps in, 178–186
    band placement, 182, 183f
    closure, 186
    dissection, 180, 181f
    port for future adjustments in, 184, 185f
    port placement, 178–180, 179f, 181f

Gastric banding, laparoscopic (*Continued*)
  pearls and pitfalls in, 186
  postoperative care in, 186
  preoperative considerations in, 177–178
  room setup and patient positioning in, 178, 179f
  surgical anatomy in, 177
Gastric bypass, Roux-en-Y, 161–176
  operative steps in, 162–172
    biliopancreatic limb in, 164
    closure, 172, 173f
    dissection into lesser sac, 164, 165f
    gastrojejunostomy creation, 170, 171f
    jejunojejunostomy creation, 164–166, 165f, 167f,
      174
    passage of Roux limb, 168, 169f
    port placement, 162, 163f
    pouch creation, 168–170, 169f, 171f, 176
  pearls and pitfalls in, 174–176
  postoperative care in, 172, 174, 176
  preoperative considerations in, 161–162, 174
  room setup and patient positioning for, 162, 163f
  surgical anatomy in, 161
Gastric conduit in esophagectomy
  in Ivor Lewis technique
    anastomosis in, 18, 19f
    creation and mobilization of, 16, 17–18
    length of, 18, 20
  laparoscopic, 36, 38
  left thoracoabdominal, 22, 24, 25f
  transhiatal, 28, 30
  tri-incisional
    creation of, 8, 9f, 13
    mobilization of, 10, 11f, 13
Gastric outlet obstruction, pyloroplasty in, 87, 97
Gastric sleeve, 187–193
Gastric veins in antrectomy, 112
Gastritis, bile reflux, 150f
Gastroduodenal artery and vein in antrectomy, 111f
Gastroduodenostomy
  in antrectomy, 110
    operative steps in, 112, 114, 124
  Jaboulay, 92, 104–109
Gastroepiploic arteries and arcade
  in antrectomy, 111f, 112, 113f
  in esophagectomy
    laparoscopic, 36
    left thoracoabdominal, 22, 26
    tri-incisional, 6, 13
  in subtotal gastrectomy, 147f, 149f
    division of, 149f
    surgical anatomy of, 145
Gastroesophageal junction
  in hiatal hernia
    paraesophageal, 52
    sliding, 40, 52
  in Nissen fundoplication, 40, 44
  tumors of
    left thoracoabdominal approach to surgery in, 21
    total gastrectomy and distal esophagectomy in,
      153
    transhiatal esophagectomy in, 27
    tri-incisional esophagectomy in, 2, 4
Gastroesophageal reflux, antireflux procedures in
  in Heller myotomy, 68–70
  in paraesophageal hernia repair, 60
Gastrohepatic ligament
  in esophagectomy
    laparoscopic, 36
    left thoracoabdominal, 22
    tri-incisional, 6
  in paraesophageal hernia
    dissection of, 56
    surgical anatomy of, 52, 54f
  in vagotomy
    highly selective, 82, 84
    selective, 80
    truncal, 74
Gastrojejunostomy
  in antrectomy, 114, 120
  in gastroparesis, postgastrectomy, 130

Gastrojejunostomy (*Continued*)
  in Roux-en-Y gastric bypass
    creation of, 170, 171f
    leaks at, 172
  truncal vagotomy with, 72
Gastroparesis, postgastrectomy, 130, 131f
Gastropexy
  in Nissen fundoplication, 48, 49f
  in paraesophageal hernia repair, 60, 61f
Gastrophrenic ligament
  in gastrectomy, total, 155f
  in vagotomy
    highly selective, 84
    selective, 80
    truncal, 74
Gastrosplenic ligament in paraesophageal hernia repair
  excessive fat from, 58, 62
  surgical anatomy of, 52, 54f
Gastrostomy
  in Finney pyloroplasty, 100, 102
  in Heineke-Mikulicz pyloroplasty, 92
    laparoscopic, 142
  in Jaboulay pyloroplasty, 108
Gastrotomy
  in antrectomy, 122
  in Jaboulay pyloroplasty, 109
  in Roux-en-Y gastric bypass, 168, 170, 171f
GIA stapler
  in esophagectomy
    Ivor Lewis, 16
    laparoscopic, 38
    tri-incisional, 8, 10, 13
  in small bowel resection and anastomosis, 194, 196
Grassi nerve
  in selective vagotomy, 79f, 80
  in truncal vagotomy, 73f, 76

H
Heineke-Mikulicz pyloroplasty, 87–95
  compared to Finney pyloroplasty, 97, 98, 103
  delayed gastric emptying after, 92
  operative steps in, 88–92
    closure, 90, 92, 93f, 94
    dissection, 88–92, 89f, 91f
    in emergent setting, 88
    Horsley modification of, 92, 93f
    identification of pylorus, 94, 95f
    incision, 87, 88, 89f, 94
    laparoscopic, 142, 143f
    traction sutures in, 88, 89f
    Weinberg modification of, 90, 91f
  pearls and pitfalls in, 94, 95f
  postoperative care in, 92
  preoperative considerations in, 87–88
  surgical anatomy in, 87
  suture line leaks in, 92, 94
Heineke-Mikulicz strictureplasty in Crohn's disease, 213–214, 215f
Heller myotomy, 65–71
  operative steps in, 65–70
    Dor fundoplication, 66, 70, 71f
    epinephrine injection, 66, 67f
    hiatal dissection, 66
    myotomy, 68, 69f
    port placement, 65
    Toupet fundoplication, 66, 68, 69f
    vagus nerves in, 66, 67f
  pearls and pitfalls in, 70
  postoperative care in, 70
  preoperative considerations in, 65
  surgical anatomy in, 65
Hepatic artery
  in antrectomy, 111f
  in paraesophageal hernia repair, 56, 62
Hepatic flexure in antrectomy, 112, 113f
Hepatoduodenal ligament in antrectomy, 115f
Hepatogastric ligament in antrectomy, 112

Hiatal hernia
  bariatric surgery in, 161, 178, 187
  Nissen fundoplication in, 40–51
  paraesophageal, 52–63
  preoperative preparations in, 40, 55
  sliding, 40, 52, 63
  types of, 52, 53f
Highly selective vagotomy, 82–86
  laparoscopic
    operative steps in, 140–142, 141f, 143f
    surgical anatomy in, 137
  operative steps in, 84, 85f
    dissection, 84, 85f
    incision, 84
    laparoscopic, 140–142, 141f, 143f
  patient positioning in, 84
  pearls and pitfalls in, 86
  postoperative care in, 86
  preoperative considerations in, 82
  surgical anatomy in, 82, 83f
    in laparoscopy, 137
  ulcer recurrence in, 86
Horsley modification of Heineke-Mikulicz pyloroplasty, 92, 93f
Hypotension, postoperative, in tri-incisional esophagectomy, 12

I
Ileocecal resection
  in Crohn's disease, laparoscopic, 218–223
    operative steps in, 218–222, 219f, 221f, 223f
    patient positioning in, 218, 219f
    pearls and pitfalls in, 222
    preoperative considerations in, 218
    room setup for, 218, 219f, 220, 221f
  in intussception, 230
Ileocolic artery in antrectomy, 111f
Ileus, postoperative, in small bowel obstruction surgery, 234
Intussception, 228–230
  indications for surgery in, 228
  laparoscopy in, 230
  in Meckel diverticulum, 224, 230
  nonoperative management of, 228
  operative steps in, 228–230, 229f
  pearls and pitfalls in, 230
  postoperative care in, 230
  preoperative considerations in, 228
  recurrence of, 230
  surgical anatomy in, 228
Ivor Lewis esophagectomy, 15–20
  advantages and disadvantages of, 15
  leaks in, 15, 18, 20
  operative steps in, 15–18
    hand-sewn anastomosis in, 18, 20
    laparotomy and gastric mobilization, 15–16
    right thoracotomy, 17–18, 19f
  pearls and pitfalls in, 20
  postoperative care in, 20
  preoperative considerations in, 15
  specimen tissue in, 17
  surgical anatomy in, 15

J
J-tube
  in Ivor Lewis esophagectomy, 16
  in laparoscopic esophagectomy, 38
  in tri-incisional esophagectomy, 10, 12
Jaboulay pyloroplasty (gastroduodenostomy), 92, 104–109
  anatomy in, 104, 105f
  delayed gastric emptying after, 108
  indications for, 104
  operative steps in, 104–108
    closure, 108
    dissection, 106, 107f

Jaboulay pyloroplasty (gastroduodenostomy) (*Continued*)
    electrocautery, 109
    in emergent setting, 104
    incision, 104–106
    traction sutures in, 106, 107f
  pearls and pitfalls in, 109
  postoperative care in, 108
  preoperative considerations in, 104
  suture line leaks in, 108
Jejunojejunostomy creation in gastric bypass, 164–166, 165f, 167f, 174
Jejunostomy, 206–212
  in antrectomy, 120
  in Finney pyloroplasty, 102
  in Heineke-Mikulicz pyloroplasty, 92
  indications for, 206
  in Jaboulay pyloroplasty, 108
  operative steps in, 206–210
  pearls and pitfalls in, 212
  permanent, 210, 211f
  postoperative care in, 210
  preoperative considerations in, 206
  replacement of tube in, 212
  Stamm-Kader technique, 208, 209f
  surgical anatomy in, 206, 207f
  volvulus of tube in, 212
  Witzel technique, 206–208, 207f, 212
Jejunum
  in antrectomy with Billroth II reconstruction, 120, 122
  in esophagectomy, laparoscopic, 38
  in jejunostomy procedures, 206–212

K
Kidneys in antrectomy, 115f
Kocher maneuver
  in antrectomy, 112
  in esophagectomy
    Ivor Lewis, 15
    laparoscopic, 36
    left thoracoabdominal, 22
    tri-incisional, 6
  in pyloroplasty
    Finney, 103
    Heineke-Mikulicz, 88
    Jaboulay, 106, 109

L
Laparoscopy
  esophagectomy in, 36–38, 37f
  gastric band placement in, 177–186
  gastric bypass in, Roux-en-Y, 161–176
  gastric ulcer surgery in, 137–144
    in gastroduodenal perforation, 138, 139f
  Heller myotomy in, 65–71
  in intussception, 230
  Nissen fundoplication in, 40–51
  paraesophageal hernia repair in, 52–63
  sleeve gastrectomy in, 187–193
  in small bowel obstruction, 234
  small bowel resection for Crohn's disease in, 218–223
  vagotomy in, 137–144
    highly selective, 137, 140–142, 141f, 143f
    truncal, and pyloroplasty, 137, 142, 143f
Laparotomy
  in Ivor Lewis esophagectomy, 15–16
  in small bowel obstruction, 231
  in transhiatal esophagectomy, 27
  in tri-incisional esophagectomy, 6, 7f
Laryngeal nerve, recurrent, in esophagectomy
  left thoracoabdominal, 24
  transhiatal, 28, 30
  tri-incisional, 1, 12, 13
Latarjet nerve
  in highly selective vagotomy, 82, 84
  in selective vagotomy, 78, 79f, 80
  in truncal vagotomy, 73f

Latissimus dorsi division and closure
  in Ivor Lewis esophagectomy, 17, 18
  in tri-incisional esophagectomy, 2, 4
Leaks
  in esophagectomy
    Ivor Lewis, 15, 18, 20
    left thoracoabdominal, 26
    tri-incisional, 12
  in gastrectomy
    subtotal, 146, 149f
    total, 159f, 160
  in gastric bypass, Roux-en-Y, 172
    intraoperative testing for, 170
    signs of, 174
  in gastric sleeve, 192
    intraoperative testing for, 190
  in pyloroplasty
    Finney, 102
    Heineke-Mikulicz, 92, 94
    Jaboulay, 108
  in small bowel resection and anastomosis, 204
Left thoracoabdominal approach to esophageal surgery,
    21–26
Lembert sutures
  in antrectomy, 116, 118, 120, 122, 124
  in Finney pyloroplasty, 100
  in Jaboulay pyloroplasty, 106
  in small bowel resection and anastomosis, 202,
    204
Liver
  in antrectomy, 112, 115f
  fatty, preparation for bariatric surgery in, 161, 178,
    187
  in paraesophageal hernia repair, 54f, 57f
    accessory left hepatic artery of, 56, 62
    in port placement, 55
  retraction of
    in antrectomy, 112
    in esophagectomy, laparoscopic, 36
    in Finney pyloroplasty, 98
    in gastric banding, laparoscopic, 177, 180
    in gastric sleeve, 188
    in Heineke-Mikulicz pyloroplasty, 88
    in Jaboulay pyloroplasty, 106
    in subtotal gastrectomy, 147f
    in total gastrectomy, 155f
    in tri-incisional esophagectomy, 6
Lymph nodes
  in esophageal cancer, dissection of, 6
  in gastric cancer
    and subtotal gastrectomy, 145, 148f
    and total gastrectomy, 155f

M
Meckel diverticulum, 224–227
  indications for surgery in, 224
  intussception in, 224, 230
  operative steps in, 224–226, 225f, 227f
  pearls and pitfalls in, 226
  preoperative considerations in, 224
  surgical anatomy in, 224
Mesenteric artery and vein in antrectomy, 111f
Mesh repair for crural closure in paraesophageal hernia,
    60
Metastasis
  esophagectomy in, tri-incisional, 6
  of gastric cancer, 145, 146
Metoprolol in tri-incisional esophagectomy, 12
Minimally invasive techniques
  in esophagectomy, 33–39
    cervical incision in, 38
    gastric conduit in, 36
    laparoscopy in, 36–38, 37f
    operative steps in, 33–38
    patient positioning in, 33, 36
    pearls and pitfalls in, 39
    port placement in, 34, 35f, 36, 37f
    postoperative care in, 39

Minimally invasive techniques (Continued)
    surgical anatomy in, 33
    thoracoscopy in, 33–34, 35f
  in gastric ulcers, 137–144
  laparoscopic. See Laparoscopy.
Motility studies of esophagus, preoperative
  in Heller myotomy, 65
  in paraesophageal hernia repair, 55
Myotomy, Heller, 65–71

N
Nasogastric intubation
  in antrectomy, 124, 126
  in Finney pyloroplasty, 97, 100, 102
  in gastric ulcer surgery, laparoscopic, 144
  in Heineke-Mikulicz pyloroplasty, 87, 92
  in Jaboulay pyloroplasty, 108
Nathanson retractor
  in gastric banding, 180, 184
  in gastric sleeve, 188
Nausea and vomiting, postoperative
  in Finney pyloroplasty, 102
  in Heineke-Mikulicz pyloroplasty, 92
  in Jaboulay pyloroplasty, 108
  in Nissen fundoplication, 50
  in paraesophageal hernia repair, 62
Nerve of Grassi
  in selective vagotomy, 79f, 80
  in truncal vagotomy, 73f, 76
Nerve of Latarjet
  in highly selective vagotomy, 82, 84
  in selective vagotomy, 78, 79f, 80
  in truncal vagotomy, 73f
Nissen-Cooper technique in antrectomy, 124
Nissen fundoplication, 40–51
  operative steps in, 40–48
    construction of wrap, 48, 49f, 51
    crural closure, 46, 47f, 51
    dissection at base of right crus, 42, 43f
    dissection of left crus, 46
    dissection of right crus, 42
    division of short gastric vessels in, 42–44, 43f, 44,
      45f, 50
    esophageal lengthening in, 46, 50
    mediastinal mobilization in, 46
    Penrose drain in, 44, 46
    port placement, 40, 41f
    posterior gastropexy, 48, 49f
  in paraesophageal hernia, 60
  pearls and pitfalls in, 50–51
  postoperative care in, 50
  preoperative considerations in, 40
  room setup in, 40, 41f
  shoe shine maneuver in, 48
  surgical anatomy in, 40
Nutrition
  in antrectomy, 110, 124
  in esophagectomy, tri-incisional, 12
  in gastrectomy
    subtotal, 146, 152
    total, 154, 159f
  in gastric banding, 178, 186
  in gastric bypass, Roux-en-Y, 161, 172, 174
  in gastric sleeve, 187, 192
  in gastric ulcer surgery, laparoscopic, 138, 144
  in Heller myotomy, 70
  in jejunostomy tube, 210
  in Nissen fundoplication, 50
  in paraesophageal hernia repair, 62
  in pyloroplasty
    Finney, 97, 102
    Heineke-Mikulicz, 87, 92
    Jaboulay, 108
  in small bowel resection and anastomosis, 204
  in vagotomy
    highly selective, 86
    selective, 80
    truncal, 76

O
Obesity surgery, 161–193
  gastric band in, 177–186
  gastric bypass in, Roux-en-Y, 161–176
  gastric sleeve in, 187–193
Obstruction
  of gastric outlet, pyloroplasty in, 87, 97
  of small intestine, 231–235. See also Small intestine,
    obstruction of.
Omentum
  in antrectomy, 111f, 112, 114, 115f, 124
  in subtotal gastrectomy, 147f, 148f
  in total gastrectomy, 156f
  in Witzel jejunostomy, 208
Omohyoid
  in transhiatal esophagectomy, 28
  in tri-incisional esophagectomy, 8
Orogastric tube
  in highly selective vagotomy, 84
  in selective vagotomy, 78
  in truncal vagotomy, 74

P
Pancreas in antrectomy
  operative steps involving, 112, 113f, 114, 115f, 116
  surgical anatomy of, 110, 111f
Pancreaticoduodenal arteries in antrectomy, 111f
Paraesophageal hernia repair, 52–63
  operative steps in, 55–60
    crural closure, 60, 61f
    fundoplication, 60
    gastropexy, 60, 61f
    hernia sac dissection, 56, 57f
    initial dissection, 56
    left crus in, 58, 59f
    mediastinal esophageal mobilization, 58, 59f, 63
    port placement, 55, 62
    right crus in, 56, 57f, 58, 59f
  pearls and pitfalls in, 62–63
  postoperative care in, 62, 63
  preoperative considerations in, 55
  surgical anatomy in, 52, 53f–54f
Parietal cell vagotomy, 82. See also Highly selective
    vagotomy.
Penrose drain
  in esophagectomy
    Ivor Lewis, 17
    laparoscopic, 38
    left thoracoabdominal, 22
    thoracoscopic, 34
    transhiatal, 28
    tri-incisional, 2, 4, 6, 8, 10
  in gastrectomy, total, 155f, 156f
  in gastric bypass, Roux-en-Y, 164
  in Heller myotomy, 66
  in Nissen fundoplication, 44, 46
  in paraesophageal hernia repair, 58
  in vagotomy, laparoscopic
    highly selective, 140
    truncal, 142
Phrenic nerve in esophagectomy
  left thoracoabdominal, 26
  tri-incisional, 6
Phrenic vein in transhiatal esophagectomy, 28
Phrenoesophageal ligament
  in Nissen fundoplication, 42, 50
  in paraesophageal hernia repair, 56
  in vagotomy
    highly selective, 84
    laparoscopic, 142
    selective, 80
    truncal, 74, 142
pH studies, esophageal
  in Heller myotomy, 65
  in paraesophageal hernia repair, 55
Platysma in esophagectomy
  laparoscopic, 38
  tri-incisional, 8, 10

Pneumatic dilatation in achalasia, 65, 70
Pneumoperitoneum
    in esophagectomy, 34, 36, 39
    in gastric ulcer surgery, 138
    in ileocecal resection for Crohn's disease, 222
    in paraesophageal hernia repair, 56
    in small bowel obstruction, 234
Portal vein in antrectomy, 111f
Port placement
    in esophagectomy
        laparoscopic, 36, 37f
        thoracoscopic, 34, 35f
    in gastric banding, 178–180, 179f, 181f
    in gastric bypass, Roux-en-Y, 162, 163f
    in gastric sleeve, 188, 189f
    in gastric ulcer surgery, 138, 139f
    in Heller myotomy, 65
    in ileocecal resection for Crohn's disease, 218, 220, 221f
    in Nissen fundoplication, 40, 41f
    in paraesophageal hernia repair, 55, 62
    in small bowel obstruction, 234
Postgastrectomy syndromes, 127–134
    afferent or efferent loop syndrome, 134, 135f
    alkaline reflux in, 132, 133f, 150f
    dumping syndrome, 127–128, 129f
    gastroparesis, 130, 131f
    preoperative considerations in, 127
    Roux stasis syndrome, 134, 135f
    surgical anatomy in, 127
Pouch creation in Roux-en-Y gastric bypass, 168–170, 169f, 171f, 176
Proton-pump inhibitor therapy
    and Finney pyloroplasty, 97
    and Heineke-Mikulicz pyloroplasty, 87, 88
Psychological evaluation in bariatric surgery
    in gastric banding, 177
    in gastric sleeve, 187
    in Roux-en-Y gastric bypass, 161, 174
Pulmonary ligament in thoracoscopic esophagectomy, 34
Pyloric vein
    in Heineke-Mikulicz pyloroplasty, 88, 89f
        laparoscopic, 142
    in subtotal gastrectomy, 149f
Pyloromyotomy
    in Ivor Lewis esophagectomy, 16
    in tri-incisional esophagectomy, 10
Pyloroplasty, 87–109
    dumping syndrome in, 127, 128, 129f
    in esophagectomy
        Ivor Lewis, 16
        laparoscopic, 36
        left thoracoabdominal, 22
        tri-incisional, 10
    Finney, 97–103
    Heineke-Mikulicz, 87–95
    Jaboulay, 104–109
    vagotomy with, 72, 87
        alkaline reflux in, 132, 133f
        dumping syndrome in, 128, 129f
        gastroparesis in, 130, 131f
        Jaboulay, 104
        laparoscopic, 137, 142, 143f
Pylorus
    identified in Heineke-Mikulicz pyloroplasty, 94, 95f
    pyloroplasty of. See Pyloroplasty.
    surgical anatomy of
        in Finney pyloroplasty, 97
        in Heineke-Mikulicz pyloroplasty, 87
        in Jaboulay pyloroplasty, 104

R
Recurrent laryngeal nerve in esophagectomy
    left thoracoabdominal, 24
    transhiatal, 28, 30
    tri-incisional, 1, 12, 13
Reflux
    alkaline, postgastrectomy, 132, 133f, 150f

Reflux (Continued)
    gastroesophageal, antireflux procedures in
        in Heller myotomy, 68–70
        in paraesophageal hernia repair, 60
Respiratory disorders, esophagectomy in
    Ivor Lewis, 15
    left thoracoabdominal, 21
    minimally invasive, 33
    transhiatal, 27
    tri-incisional, 2
Roux-en-Y anastomosis
    in esophagectomy, left thoracoabdominal, 21
    in esophagojejunostomy and total gastrectomy, 157f–159f
    in gastric bypass, 161–176
    in postgastrectomy syndromes
        in alkaline reflux, 132, 133f
        in dumping, 128, 129f
        in gastroparesis, 130, 131f
    stasis syndrome in, 134, 135f
Roux stasis syndrome, postgastrectomy, 134, 135f

S
Schofield retractors in gastric banding, 184, 186
Selective vagotomy, 78–81
    highly selective, 82–86
    laparoscopic, 137
    operative steps in, 78–80, 81f
        dissection, 80, 81f
        incision, 78
    patient positioning in, 78
    pearls and pitfalls in, 80
    postoperative care in, 80
    preoperative considerations in, 78
    surgical anatomy in, 78, 79f, 80, 137
Shoe shine maneuver in Nissen fundoplication, 48
Sleeve gastrectomy, 187–193
    indications for, 187, 192
    operative steps in, 188–192, 189f, 191f, 193f
    pearls and pitfalls in, 192
    port placement in, 188, 189f
    postoperative care in, 192
    preoperative considerations in, 187–188
    room setup and patient positioning in, 188, 189f
    surgical anatomy in, 187
Sliding hiatal hernia, 40, 52, 63
Small intestine, 194–235
    Crohn's disease of, 213–223
        laparoscopic resection in, 218–223
        strictureplasty in, 213–217
    duodenum. See Duodenum.
    intussusception of, 228–230
    jejunostomy tube, 206–212
    jejunum. See Jejunum.
    Meckel diverticulum of, 224–227
    obstruction of, 231–235
        laparoscopy in, 234, 235f
        open resection in, 231–232, 233f
        pearls and pitfalls in, 234
        postoperative care in, 234
        preoperative considerations in, 231
    resection and anastomosis of, 194–205
        hand-sewn anastomosis, 194, 198–204, 199f, 201f, 203f, 205f
        in intussusception, 228, 230
        laparoscopic, in Crohn's disease, 218–223
        in Meckel diverticulum, 224, 226
        in obstruction, 231–232, 233f
        pearls and pitfalls in, 204
        postoperative care in, 204
        preoperative considerations in, 194
        stapled anastomosis, 194–196, 195f, 197f
Smoking cessation, preoperative
    in gastric banding, 177
    in gastric bypass, Roux-en-Y, 161
    in gastric sleeve, 187
Specimen tissue
    in esophagectomy

Specimen tissue (Continued)
    Ivor Lewis, 17
    left thoracoabdominal, 24
    tri-incisional, 2, 4, 8
    in gastrectomy
        subtotal, 150f
        total, 157f
    in ileocecal resection for Crohn's disease, 222
Spleen
    in antrectomy, 110, 111f, 115f
    in gastrectomy
        subtotal, 152
        total, 156f
    in gastric banding, laparoscopic, 180
Stamm-Kader jejunostomy, 208, 209f
Stapling techniques
    in antrectomy, 114, 116, 122, 126
    in esophagectomy
        Ivor Lewis, 16, 18
        laparoscopic, 36, 38
        left thoracoabdominal, 22
        tri-incisional, 8, 10, 13
    in gastrectomy
        subtotal, 150f
        total, 157f–158f
    in gastric bypass, Roux-en-Y
        in gastrojejunostomy creation, 170, 171f
        in jejunojejunostomy creation, 164, 166, 174
        in pouch creation, 168–170
    in gastric sleeve, 190, 191f
    in Meckel diverticulectomy, 226, 227f
    in pyloroplasty, Heineke-Mikulicz, 92, 93f
    in small bowel resection and anastomosis, 194–196, 195f, 197f
Sternocleidomastoid muscle in transhiatal esophagectomy, 28
Stomach
    antrectomy of, 110–126
    bariatric surgery of, 161–193
    cancer surgery of, 145–160
    delayed emptying of
        in Finney pyloroplasty, 102
        in Heineke-Mikulicz pyloroplasty, 92
        in Jaboulay pyloroplasty, 108
        in paraesophageal hernia repair, 63
        postgastrectomy, 130, 131f
    in esophagectomy
        as conduit. See Gastric conduit in esophagectomy.
        Ivor Lewis, 15, 16, 17–18, 20
        laparoscopic, 36
        left thoracoabdominal, 21
        tri-incisional, 1, 6, 8, 9f, 10, 11f, 13
    in fundoplication procedures. See Fundoplication.
    gastrectomy of, 145–160
    gastropexy techniques
        in Nissen fundoplication, 48, 49f
        in paraesophageal hernia repair, 60, 61f
    in Heller myotomy, 65
        and Dor fundoplication, 66, 70, 71f
        and Toupet fundoplication, 66, 68, 69f
    increased emptying of, postgastrectomy, 127–128
    in paraesophageal hernia repair
        in fundoplication, 60
        in gastropexy, 60, 61f
        postoperative delayed emptying of, 63
        retraction for initial dissection, 56
        surgical anatomy of, 52, 54f
    pyloroplasty of, 87–109. See also Pyloroplasty.
    surgical anatomy of
        in antrectomy, 110, 111f
        in gastric banding, 177
        in paraesophageal hernia repair, 52, 54f
        in subtotal gastrectomy, 145
        in total gastrectomy, 153
        in tri-incisional esophagectomy, 1
    thermal injury in Nissen fundoplication, 42, 44
    ulcer disease of
        antrectomy in, 110, 114
        laparoscopic surgery in, 137–144
    vagotomy procedures of, 72–86

Strictureplasty in Crohn's disease, 213–217
  contraindications to, 216
  indications for, 213
  operative steps in, 213–217
    in Finney technique, 216, 217f
    in Heineke-Mikulicz technique, 213–214, 215f
  pearls and pitfalls in, 216
  preoperative considerations in, 213
  surgical anatomy in, 213
Subclavian artery in left thoracoabdominal
    esophagectomy, 21, 26
Subtotal gastrectomy, 145–152
  contraindications to, 147f
  operative steps in, 146, 147f–151f
    anastomosis in, 151f, 152
    gastric arteries in, 147f, 148f, 152
    in lymph node involvement, 148f
    roux limb in, 151f
    surgical margins in, 150f
  pearls and pitfalls in, 152
  postoperative care in, 152
  preoperative considerations in, 145–146
  specimen tissue in, 150f
  surgical anatomy in, 145

T
Thoracic duct in esophagectomy
  left thoracoabdominal, 21
    injury of, 24, 26
  tri-incisional, 4, 5f
    injury of, 4, 12
Thoracoabdominal approach to esophageal surgery, left,
    21–26
  leaks in, 26
  operative steps in, 22–24, 23f, 25f
  patient positioning in, 22
  pearls and pitfalls in, 26
  postoperative care in, 26
  preoperative considerations in, 21
  specimen tissue in, 24
  surgical anatomy in, 21
Thoracoscopic esophagectomy, 33–34, 35f
Thoracotomy in esophagectomy
  Ivor Lewis, 17–18, 19f
  left thoracoabdominal, 22
  tri-incisional, 2–4, 3f, 5f
Thromboembolism prevention
  in Finney pyloroplasty, 97
  in gastric banding, 186
  in gastric bypass, Roux-en-Y, 162, 172
  in gastric sleeve, 188, 192
  in Heineke-Mikulicz pyloroplasty, 88
  in tri-incisional esophagectomy, 1, 12
Thyroid vein in transhiatal esophagectomy, 28
Total gastrectomy, 153–160
  indications for, 145, 146, 150f
  operative steps in, 154, 155f–159f
    anastomosis in, 154, 156f, 157f–159f, 160
    surgical margins in, 155f, 157f
  pearls and pitfalls in, 160
  postoperative care in, 154
  preoperative considerations in, 153, 160
  surgical anatomy in, 153
Toupet fundoplication
  in Heller myotomy, 66, 68, 69f
  in paraesophageal hernia, 60
Trachea
  intubation in total gastrectomy, 153
  in thoracoscopic esophagectomy, 34
  in transhiatal esophagectomy, 28, 29f, 30, 32

Transhiatal esophagectomy, 27–32
  indications for, 27
  operative steps in, 27–30, 29f, 31f
    cervical anastomosis, 30
    cervical incision, 28, 29f
    dissection, 28–30, 29f, 32
    gastric conduit in, 28, 30
  patient positioning in, 27
  pearls and pitfalls in, 32
  postoperative care in, 30
  surgical anatomy in, 27
Tri-incisional esophagectomy, 1–13
  advantages and disadvantages of, 2
  leaks in, 12
  operative steps in, 2–10
    cervical phase, 8–10, 9f, 11f
    laparotomy, 6, 7f
    pyloroplasty or pyloromyotomy, 10
    right thoracotomy, 2–4, 3f, 5f
  patient positioning in, 2
  pearls and pitfalls in, 13
  postoperative care in, 12
  preoperative considerations in, 1–2
  specimen tissue in, 2, 4, 8
  surgical anatomy in, 1
Truncal vagotomy, 72–77
  with antrectomy, 72, 86, 110
    alkaline reflux in, 132, 133f
    dumping syndrome in, 128, 129f
    gastroparesis in, 130, 131f
    laparoscopic, 137
  laparoscopic, 137, 142, 143f
  operative steps in, 72–75
    dissection, 74, 75f
    incision, 72
    laparoscopic, 142, 143f
  patient positioning in, 72, 74
  pearls and pitfalls in, 76
  postoperative care in, 76
  preoperative considerations in, 72
  with pyloroplasty
    alkaline reflux in, 132, 133f
    dumping syndrome in, 128
    gastroparesis in, 130, 131f
    Jaboulay, 104
    laparoscopic, 137, 142, 143f
  surgical anatomy in, 72, 73f
    in laparoscopy, 137
Tumors
  of esophagus
    Ivor Lewis esophagectomy in, 15–20
    left thoracoabdominal approach to, 21–26
    minimally invasive esophagectomy in, 33–39
    transhiatal esophagectomy in, 27–32
    tri-incisional esophagectomy in, 1–13
  of gastroesophageal junction. See Gastroesophageal
    junction, tumors of.
  of stomach, 145–160
    antrectomy in, 110
    metastasis of, 145, 146
    preoperative evaluation of, 145–146, 152, 153, 155f,
      160
    subtotal gastrectomy in, 145–152
    total gastrectomy in, 145, 146, 150f, 153–160

U
Ulcer disease
  antrectomy in, 110, 115f
    operative steps in, 112, 114, 118, 124
  Finney pyloroplasty in, 97, 103

Ulcer disease (Continued)
  Heineke-Mikulicz pyloroplasty in, 87, 92, 93f
  Jaboulay pyloroplasty and truncal vagotomy in,
    104
  laparoscopic surgery in, 137–144
    in gastroduodenal perforation, 138, 139f, 144
    indications for, 137–138
    operative steps in, 138–144
    pearls and pitfalls in, 144
    postoperative care in, 144
    preoperative considerations in, 137–138
    surgical anatomy in, 137
  vagotomy in. See Vagotomy.

V
Vagotomy, 72–86
  with antrectomy. See Antrectomy, vagotomy with.
  highly selective, 82–86. See also Highly selective
    vagotomy.
  laparoscopic, 137–144
    operative steps in, 140–144
    pearls and pitfalls in, 144
    postoperative care in, 144
    preoperative considerations in, 137–138
    surgical anatomy in, 137
  with pyloroplasty. See Pyloroplasty, vagotomy with.
  selective, 78–81. See also Selective vagotomy.
  truncal, 72–77, 86. See also Truncal vagotomy.
  ulcer recurrence in, 86
Vagus nerve
  in esophagectomy
    Ivor Lewis, 17
    thoracoscopic, 34
    in tri-incisional, 2, 13
  in gastric bypass, Roux-en-Y, 168
  in Heller myotomy, 66, 67f
  in Nissen fundoplication, 46
  in paraesophageal hernia repair, 58, 63
  surgical anatomy of
    in highly selective vagotomy, 82, 83f
    in laparoscopic vagotomy, 137
    in selective vagotomy, 78, 79f, 80
    in total gastrectomy, 153
    in truncal vagotomy, 72, 73f
  vagotomy of. See Vagotomy.
Video barium swallow, preoperative, in paraesophageal
  hernia repair, 55

W
Weinberg modification of Heineke-Mikulicz pyloroplasty,
  90, 91f
Witzel jejunostomy, 206–208, 207f, 212

X
Xiphoid process
  in Finney pyloroplasty incision, 98
  in gastric banding port placement, 178
  in gastric bypass port placement, 162
  in gastric sleeve port placement, 188
  in Heineke-Mikulicz pyloroplasty incision, 88
  in Jaboulay pyloroplasty incision, 104
  in tri-incisional esophagectomy, 6